WHAT IN THE BABY?!?

THE MODERN MAMA'S GUIDE TO CONFIDENTLY CARING FOR YOUR BABY AND SURVIVING THE POSTPARTUM PERIOD

Mercedes Thomas, CPNP, IBCLC

Copyright © 2020 by Mercedes Thomas.
All rights reserved.

No part of this publication may be reproduced, stored in a retrieval system, or transmitted in any form or by any means including photocopying, recording, or other electronic or mechanical methods, written, electronic, or without written permission of the author, except for the brief quotations in a book review. Any inquiries relating to this publication or author may be emailed to hello@mercedesthomas.com.

The contents of this book are for informational purposes only and not meant to serve as a substitute for the professional medical or dietary advice of you or your child's healthcare provider.
No liability is assumed for damages that may result from the use of the information contained within.

To ensure confidentiality, all patient and client names within this book are not the real names of patients cared for at any point in time. All stories in this book have been modified to protect privacy.

Published by:
Thomas Health Education and Consulting, LLC
ISBN: 978-1-7354664-0-8

Contents

Introduction 1

CHAPTER 1: Preparing for Baby 5

CHAPTER 2: The Fourth Trimester 21

CHAPTER 3: Baby Care & Tips 33

CHAPTER 4: Adapting to Motherhood 45

CHAPTER 5: Breastfeeding & Bottle Feeding 55

CHAPTER 6: Infant Safety & Health 75

CHAPTER 7: Explaining Facts vs. Myths 89

CHAPTER 8: Sleep & Developmental Milestones 97

Closing Thoughts 107

Acknowledgments 109

APPENDIX A: Resources 111

APPENDIX B: References 117

Introduction

Welcome, I'm Mercedes, the author of *What in the Baby?!?*™: *The Modern Mama's Guide to Confidently Caring for Your Baby and Surviving the Postpartum Period*. I'm so excited that you've chosen my book to help you learn all about baby care and to prepare for your transition into motherhood. I created this book with mamas just like you in mind.

It wasn't until my rite of passage into motherhood that I had a compelling need to finally turn my idea for this book into a reality. The idea for this book isn't a new one; in fact, until the summer of 2020, it lived in a Microsoft Word document that I created at the beginning of my nursing career. Why? Simply put, motherhood isn't easy; it's beautiful, amazing, even crazy at times, and can be full of surprises, but easy isn't a word that I've ever heard used to describe it. So it was my hope to create a guide to help modern mamas prepare for their baby and empower themselves with reputable information that was easy to understand without a bunch of fluff. As you continue reading, you'll find tips and topics that are important as you transition to the new normal of motherhood. These topics include baby care, infant safety, the fourth trimester, postpartum depression, breastfeeding, bottle feeding, developmental milestones, sleep, and much more!

You might be thinking, how is this book different from all the other baby books out there? My answer is that it's different in many ways because this book was written specifically for modern and millennial moms, using over a decade of pediatric and neonatal nursing knowledge that I've acquired and my personal experience as a mom.

I'll share stories with you and helpful lists that will allow you to have something to refer back to but most importantly, I bring you the evidence. Yes, the evidence! You know, facts and scientific proof to back it up! Sure, my professional and personal opinion matters, but in an age of "it worked for me," we all soon learn that what worked for your neighbor or your friend in the local mom group may not work for you or your baby.

Although this book is written in "my voice," telling only the stories that I could tell, it was important to me that I provided you with interesting tips that are easy to read. I wanted to do this without all the long, hard to understand words that healthcare providers sometimes use.

I've made it a point to include many of the baby-related topics that I've come across working with patients and parents over the last decade. Which consists of the things that come up the most in conversation and during the parenting classes that I teach. As you read through this book, you'll find the answers to many of the questions that I'm frequently asked by parents and those topics that I see new mamas struggle with the most. To be perfectly honest, I've included many things that I've even struggled with as a new mama too! Also, in Appendix A, I've included a comprehensive list of resources that you can refer back to at any time.

Even though I'm a pediatric nurse practitioner and now an International Board Certified Lactation Consultant (IBCLC), I'm human and didn't have the perfect transition into motherhood, especially when it came time to breastfeed my son. Since the immediate postpartum period is such a time of vulnerability, sleepless nights, and quite frankly a real adjustment, *What in the Baby?!?*™ focuses heavily on the fourth trimester, which starts right after your baby is born up until around twelve weeks postpartum.

As you begin reading *What in the Baby?!?*™, you'll see that the first letter of the title in chapters three through eight spells out "BABIES." The B.A.B.I.E.S Method™ is a system that I created to teach moms like you what they truly need to know to start on their parenting journey.

The acronym **B.A.B.I.E.S** stand for:
- **B**aby care & tips
- **A**dapting to motherhood
- **B**reast & bottle feeding
- **I**nfant safety & health
- **E**xplaining Facts vs. Myths
- **S**leep & developmental milestones

I found coming up with acronyms and mnemonics back when I was in nursing school to be one of my favorite ways to remember complex material. I hope you like some of the ones that I've included throughout the book, especially for you. This book isn't a nursing exam, and I'm sure you're happy about that. As a new mama, I know you want and need straightforward, easy-to-remember tips that you can use and won't strain your brain.

Last but not least, the advocate in me never sleeps. I want you to know that another reason that this book exists is to help improve health outcomes with the purpose of "fighting" against infant and maternal health disparities (poor health outcomes) for mamas and babies across the globe. We all deserve better when it comes to the care of our bodies by healthcare providers, not to mention our emotions as we step out into the world as mothers because mental health is just as important as physical health. By educating yourself through books, classes, and reputable resources in your community (online or locally), I believe that you're able to take back the power to live your best mom life!

Now I want you to relax in your favorite chair or bed and put your parenting anxieties aside and figure out *What in the Baby?!?*™ you need to know as you gear up to give motherhood a go!

Thank you for trusting me to be a resource as you embark on the journey of welcoming your tiny bundle of joy!

Peace, happiness & wellness!
Mercedes Thomas, CPNP, IBCLC
www.MercedesThomas.com

CHAPTER 1

Preparing for Your Baby

*"Being a parent is like folding a fitted sheet;
no one really knows how."*

—UNKNOWN

Even though I have over 12 years of experience in pediatric and neonatal nursing (think babies who were born too early), I felt that taking a childbirth class would be a great way to help prepare my husband and I for the birth of our baby. After some discussion with my husband, we decided to take a weekend childbirth class series. Boy, was I glad because I was filled with worry thinking that he may be "that husband" during the delivery of our baby boy! What does "that husband" mean, you ask? Well, to me, it would be the stereotypical husband that we have all seen in a movie who faints. I mean, let's face it, my husband caring for me while sick with a cold is a far cry from stomaching blood, bodily fluids, and potentially uncontrollable screaming while laboring. So I was left wondering how he might react. Just in case you're wondering, he did a fantastic job supporting me and didn't even come close to passing out.

Anyway, I'll get back to the topic at hand, which is childbirth education. We opted to take a group class at the hospital that I planned to deliver at, and it was great. Our instructor had been a nurse for a gazillion years, so she had a ton of professional experience. In addition to being a certified childbirth educator, she was also an International Board Certified Lactation Consultant (IBCLC) – I'll talk more about what that means in Chapter 5, which is all about breast and bottle feeding. I mean, who wouldn't love taking a class where your husband gets taught how to massage and coach you through labor while listening to lullabies to the tune of popular songs?

In hindsight, because we were so busy and working full-time, it would've been nice to have the option to take some or all of the childbirth class virtually. Hence, the reason why I decided to offer virtual classes and workshops to parents in my private practice. My experiences while pregnant and as a new mom have shaped the way I currently practice, and for that, I'm very grateful.

Education is the Key

The best thing you can do for yourself as an expectant or new mom to prepare is to take a class or two. The great thing is that nowadays, there are so many options for courses that will teach you everything you ever wanted to know about caring for your baby. Even if you've never had the experience of being on baby duty, there are classes you can take that can walk you through how to feed your baby by breast or bottle. If you feel like you need to learn basic baby care like swaddling a baby or the steps to changing a diaper, there's a class for that. Believe me, doing so is a science, especially if you've never changed a baby boy's diaper. Think water fountain, and you'll catch my drift! You should also consider taking a class on infant safety to learn how to perform cardiopulmonary resuscitation (CPR) and intervene if choking were to occur.

Let's talk format. Depending on how you learn best or your preferences, there is something to fit you and your partner's needs. Some of the most common options include are in-person or virtual classes that you can take in a group with other parents. If you prefer more of an intimate setting, private in-home classes are also a thing. You may wonder how in the world you can learn hands-on skills like diapering, swaddling, or even feeding your baby if you opt for a virtual class? Well, the answer is straightforward. For example, I use videos while teaching live virtual classes, do demonstrations with my favorite teaching doll Miles, and use breast and bottle props to provide visuals. Another perk is that if you purchase a recorded virtual class, you can watch it again later, which is a great way to review some of the skills or topics you'd like a little more practice with before or after your baby is born.

Educating yourself is essential because it helps decrease some of the natural anxieties associated with becoming a new mom. Even though I talked about classes that you can take to prepare for your bundle of joy already, I also want to point out that there are many great e-books or paperback books—if you prefer to still turn the pages like back in the good 'ole days. Books like this one, of course, shameless plug, I know, but I figured why not since you're already reading it anyway.

Childbirth Classes

There are several types of classes you may want to consider taking. My recommendation is to just focus on a couple as not to overwhelm yourself. My top picks are childbirth classes, where you can learn all about the birthing process and more about what to expect. Childbirth is like no other experience I've had as a woman and mom. It was the most beautiful, crazy, fantastic event of my life mixed with a side of pain (ouch!), but it was worth it.

You can choose to get specific with childbirth education, like taking a class to prepare for and learn more about natural childbirth or homebirth. You could even take a hypnobirthing class to learn relaxation techniques and how to positively channel your thoughts in preparation for birth. I don't have personal experience with hypnobirthing methods, but I have heard many positive reviews from my clients and colleagues.

I recommend that you do a little research and see what may work best for you. Also, it's a great idea to have your partner or support person of choice attend any classes with you. If you don't have a support person, or even if you do, looking into hiring a doula is a great idea, and I'll talk more about that later on in this chapter.

The Birth Plan

Besides learning about the birthing process, taking a quality childbirth education class should provide you with the basic knowledge to start planning for your own birth. A written or electronic copy of your birth plan is usually the most common way to communicate your preferences. A birth plan should be used as a guide and is an excellent way for you to participate in shared decision-making with your healthcare provider. However, it may need to be tweaked based on you or your baby's medical history or situations that may

occur during or after your baby is born. You can find a template online, make one yourself, or ask your childbirth education instructor for resources (see Appendix A for further information).

Breastfeeding Classes

Did you think that I would let you read on without stressing the importance of taking a prenatal breastfeeding class? Nope, not a chance! As a lactation consultant and breastfeeding advocate who breastfed my son for over two years, I have to tell you that taking a breastfeeding class is so important no matter who you are.

Research shows that women who have support during their breastfeeding journeys are more likely to breastfeed longer and continue to persevere even if they encounter a couple of "bumps in the road." Why? One of the primary reasons is they can learn all of the basics in a relaxed setting and ask questions that can prevent them from becoming discouraged early on if breastfeeding doesn't turn out to be as effortless as expected. Again, I recommend selecting a class that best fits your lifestyle and preferred mode of learning. Those options range from taking an online course, one at your local hospital, and even purchasing books to supplement your learning.

La Leche League International (LLLI) is also a great free resource offering local support groups that you can attend prenatally and after your baby is born, depending on where you live. There is also a wealth of evidence-based information on their website. Again, no matter the type of class you choose, I encourage you to have your partner or support person attend so that they can learn the basics about breastfeeding as well.

Some topics that you can expect to review in your prenatal breastfeeding class include:
- The benefits of breastfeeding
- Common myths
- What to expect in the first hours and days after birth
- Positioning and latching tips
- How to know if your baby is getting enough milk

CHAPTER 1: **Preparing for Your Baby** 11

- How to establish and maintain a good milk supply
- Feeding cues
- Common pitfalls and how to avoid them – this is a big one!!
- How to find evidence-based breastfeeding information you can trust.
- How to get help and support with breastfeeding when you need it.

Your Support System
Family and Friends

Being a new mother is so amazing and beautiful, but that doesn't negate the fact that it's also an adjustment, so it's a good idea to line up help from family and friends if you can. We personally didn't have any family nearby after I had my son. My mother and mother-in-law both live pretty far away, so they had to book flights to visit. We decided to stagger their visits on purpose to have help for an extended period of time, and boy was I grateful for this plan.

My mother and mother-in-law were able to cook and prepare meals, help clean the house, wash clothing, and help me with the baby so that I could do important things like shower and get a little more rest. If possible, it's a great idea to prepare meals and freeze them before your baby is born. Cue up your Pinterest app and find some quick, easy recipes that freeze well. Trust me, you'll be so happy you did.

The Scoop on Doulas

If you don't have a support system or even if you do right down the street, one thing to consider as a new mom is hiring a doula. What is a doula, you ask?

According to DONA International, a doula is a "trained professional who provides continuous physical, emotional, and informational support to a mother before, during, and shortly after childbirth to help her achieve the healthiest, most satisfying experience possible." [1] If you feel like hiring a doula may be a good fit for you and your family, start interviewing early on. You can find an independent doula or one that works as part of an agency; the choice is up to you.

If you're not sure how to find a doula, an excellent place to start is by asking your network of mommy friends, family, your healthcare provider, or try asking in a local mom group. Another great resource where you can read reviews is the Doula Match website (see Appendix A). There are two common types of doulas that most parents decide upon. Birth doulas usually help support you from around the third trimester of your pregnancy through the first couple of hours after the birth of your baby. Postpartum doulas help families after the birth of their baby with support services that include caring for the newborn and helping with household duties like cooking, prepping meals, light housekeeping, or tending to older siblings.

CHAPTER 1: **Preparing for Your Baby**

Preparing the Nursery

Will you go with the classic pink or blue? To paint or not to paint? Will you go for trendy, gender-neutral, modern, or just keep it simple? There are so many decisions to make when deciding what type of nursery you'll pick for your new baby (or babies, yay multiples). My recommendation is to start brainstorming and work on having the most important items ready and put together around 1 to 2 months before your expected due date. The following items are a good place to start:

- The crib – skip the bumpers because they're unsafe. Also, be sure to review the manufacturer's safety guidelines and search for recalls on the crib(s) you're considering before purchasing
- A rocking chair
- Changing table
- A dresser for storing clothing

Stocking Up On The Essentials

If you've opted to create a baby registry, you may receive most of what you need from family and friends, and that's truly a blessing. Or maybe you've opted not to have one. Either way, I created a list of staple items that you'll want to have on hand before your baby arrives.

The Supplies:

- Diapers
- Diaper cream
- Wipes
- Tylenol – it's good to have on hand, but please only use this under the direction of your child's primary care provider as this isn't generally recommended for a newborn. I'll talk more about safety guidelines in Chapter 6.
- Laundry detergent – try to stick to free and clear detergents that are unscented because they are less likely to irritate your baby's skin.
- A thermometer – to take your newborn's temperature rectally.

Clothing Items:

- Onesies and sleepers, depending on the season and the temperature in your home. A comfortable temperature for many is around 70 to 72 degrees Fahrenheit. The rule of thumb is to dress your baby in no more than one extra layer of clothing than you would typically wear. This will help to prevent him or her from getting too warm.
- Avoid the urge to buy a ton of newborn-sized clothes. Babies tend to grow pretty quickly, and you'll want to have a variety of sizes.

- Consider that you'll need at least 2 to 3 changes of clothes per day for the first month or so because, let's face it, baby clothes can get soiled with poop, urine, milk, or spit-up at any given time.

Packing Your Hospital (Or Birth Center) Bag

Around 3 to 4 weeks before your due date is a great time to pack your bag (unless you're planning on having a home birth) and maybe even your partner's if they're procrastinating. When they're ready to make their debut in the world, babies don't wait, and the last thing you want is to be scrambling to pack the essentials at the last minute. If you're anything like me and want the bag packed with particular items, you want time to do it yourself instead of leaving it up to your beloved partner to blindly figure it out because you're already at the hospital. *smiles*

If I had one piece of advice for you, it would be to not overdo it. Now, if you're not a minimalist like me, this may be a challenging task. Until I recently found a new mom to donate them to, I still had the monster-sized sanitary pads leftover in my bathroom cabinet from when I had my son in 2018. So, take it from me and don't go overboard because most of the supplies you'll need will be provided to you at the hospital.

Here Are Some of The Essentials You Should Plan on Packing:

- Your hospital paperwork, a picture ID (like your driver's license), and your health insurance card.
- Comfy, stretchy sleepwear and underwear to wear in the hospital and come home in because despite what those celeb moms may look like, it will take the typical woman several weeks to months to drop the pregnancy weight. I mean, after all, it took 9 months to gain it, so give yourself some grace.
- Your personal toiletries like a toothbrush, toothpaste, lip balm, soap, comb, brush, and hair ties. I think you get the point.
- Slippers or socks – go with something that has a non-slip sole, or you may just opt to use the socks available at the hospital.
- An outfit for your baby to wear home and blanket(s). Now, remember when I said I wasn't a minimalist? Well, I sprung for the cute matching hat and sleeper with my son's initials and name on it. You don't have to do this, but this is a great way to get some great pictures before leaving the hospital for your memory book.
- A robe – spring for the nice soft, comfy one even if it isn't trendy. See the theme here? You won't regret choosing comfort over cute.

- Your own pillow(s) because you may need five of the pancake-flat ones in the hospital to come close to your favorite plush one from home. Shhhh, don't tell the hospital staff our little secret.
- A scarf. If this went over your head, don't worry about it, but some of us mamas may need it to protect or maintain our hair.
- Chargers for your electronic devices.
- A good book or two and magazines.

Selecting a Pediatrician or a Pediatric Nurse Practitioner (PNP) For Your Baby

Choosing the right healthcare provider for your child is one of the most important decisions you'll make in preparing for the birth of your baby.

Insider tip: Arrange for a prenatal visit where you can go visit local pediatric offices and interview potential pediatricians or pediatric nurse practitioners (PNPs) like me. Note that these tours may not be available in person regularly during or after the COVID-19 pandemic era, but a phone or video meeting may be a good alternative to consider.

Many people know that a pediatrician is a doctor who specializes in caring for children. However, you may not be familiar with PNPs, so I'd like to give a quick overview of our role. Simply put, a pediatric nurse practitioner is a registered nurse who obtained a master's or doctoral degree and completed a minimum of 500 hours directly caring for pediatric patients. In most cases, pediatric patients range from newborn to 21 years of age. PNPs can also write prescriptions, order labs and diagnostic tests in addition to the ability to diagnose. Depending on the state, PNPs may need to collaborate with a physician to practice, but in full practice states like Maryland, where I'm currently licensed, we can practice independently. Well, that was a mouthful now, wasn't it? I just wanted to make sure it was clear that you have different options when choosing your child's primary care provider.

Now let's get to the heart of this section, which is a list of potential questions that you can use to interview a pediatrician or PNP to help you decide if they would be a good fit to take care of your baby. The following questions cover the basics:

1. Will you come to the hospital to see my baby after he or she is born? Note: Often, the doctor(s) on call will care for all newborns born while they're working their shift. Some providers work in pediatric offices and go into the hospital to visit and examine their patients after they're born.

2. Are you board certified? What are your qualifications?

3. Is the way that you practice similar to your colleagues who also work in the same office?

4. Will my baby be able to see the same provider at every visit?

CHAPTER 1: **Preparing for Your Baby** 19

5. Do you follow the most current and up-to-date guidelines from the American Academy of Pediatrics (AAP)? This is a great question to gauge whether your doctor practices using evidence-based information.

6. How do you support breastfeeding mothers? Do you have any additional training or certifications related to lactation?

7. What are your views on vaccines, circumcision, infant sleep, and antibiotics usage?

8. If I have a question or concern after hours, is there an on-call provider that I can call to speak with?

9. Are same day appointments available if my baby is ill?

10. What health insurance plans does your office accept?

11. Do you have any other pediatric healthcare professionals that work in your office? Some examples would be a lactation consultant, a speech therapist, or a physical therapist.

12. Does your waiting room have a separate area for sick and well children? This helps to keep children that a sick from spreading germs to those who are not.

CHAPTER 2

The Fourth Trimester

"Being a mom has made me so tired and so happy."
—TINA FEY

On an early spring morning, Samantha and her husband Jeff arrived at my office for baby Jenna's second check-up around one month after she was born. Samantha's hair was up in a loose bun, and she was wearing leggings and a cute floral dress. Jeff was in sweat pants and a t-shirt and smiling from ear to ear like a proud father. I remember that this was one of my first appointments of the day because, in pediatrics, we generally like to get our tiniest patients scheduled first thing in the morning so they can avoid the crowds that usually come in the afternoon once school and work let out.

Samantha seemed happy, but I could tell she was slightly frazzled as she tried to rock and comfort baby Jenna, who was screaming and crying after being examined by me… oopsie! Jeff scrambled to help Samantha dress baby Jenna and help to settle her. With all of the commotion in the background, I read over Samantha's Edinburgh, a questionnaire formally referred to as the Edinburgh Postnatal Depression Scale (EDPS), which is used to screen mothers for potential signs of postpartum depression.

Samantha's answers on the questionnaire didn't indicate that she was suffering from depression.

However, her score, coupled with our conversation during baby Jenna's visit, alerted me that she was struggling some and could probably use additional support services. We openly talked about my findings, and she agreed that she would be happy to accept some recommendations for community referrals. I provided Samantha with reassurance and a list of resources that she could access. With Samantha's permission, I also contacted her primary care provider so that he would be aware and follow up with her.

Fast forward to baby Jenna's two-month visit, where Samantha showed up in better spirits and more confident as a new mother. For Samantha, this was a happy ending. However, it's not uncommon for some new mothers to require much closer follow-up due to the intense emotions that they experience after giving birth. Frequently the emotions experienced are linked to postpartum hormone changes. Some mothers may need immediate help like a mental health professional referral for further evaluation and treatment.

The Fourth Trimester Transition

I'd like to start by highlighting that your pregnancy is broken up into three trimesters, each associated with countless guidelines and defining milestones from conception to birth. However, the immediate period after having a baby is just as important but often overlooked in the information

CHAPTER 2: **The Fourth Trimester** 23

available to new moms. So, let's get to the point of this chapter, which is to explain the details of the fourth trimester so that you can be prepared for what may lay ahead.

The fourth trimester isn't a new term, but perhaps you're staring at the page with a blank stare, wondering what in the world I'm talking about. Simply put, the fourth trimester starts from the time that your baby is born and encompasses the 12 weeks that immediately follow your baby's birth. The first three months after having a baby is a timeframe when most women are at their most vulnerable point. This may be especially true after family and friends get back to their lives after the initial celebration of the new baby and mom. To make matters even worse when it comes to figuring it all out, your first check-up with your doctor is usually not until six weeks from the date you gave birth.

The Nitty Gritty On Life After Birth
Skin to Skin

Let's start from the very beginning after you've had your little one. You've pushed and maybe screamed some depending on how you felt during your birth. Once your baby is born, your OB-GYN or midwife will usually place your baby on your chest because it's time for you or your partner to cut the umbilical cord.

Now, did you catch the part about you cutting the cord? Um yeah, so back to my hubby, who you "met" briefly in the first chapter; he wasn't exactly thrilled about cutting our son's umbilical cord, so in regular Mercedes fashion, I took the challenge and cut it myself. Anyway, I digress, back to the minutes just after your provider puts your brand new baby onto your chest.

I highly recommend skin-to-skin, which is the act of having your baby lay completely unclothed up against your bare skin. Skin-to-skin is where the magic happens, and research proves it. Skin-to-skin facilitates bonding immediately and helps regulate your baby's temperature, just to name a few benefits. Not to mention that lovely "golden hour," which is the first 60 minutes after giving birth where your baby is usually the most alert and if you've opted to breastfeed, he or she is ready to find his or her way to your breast to do just that. Skin-to-skin is also a great way to get your partner involved and allow time to bond with your bundle of joy. Later on, in Chapter 5, I'll talk more in-depth about feeding your baby.

Postpartum Wishes

One of the best things you can do in preparing for the fourth trimester is to plan and then communicate your plan. Yes, I know there goes the "p-word" again. Still, one of the most helpful ways to decrease unnecessary stress and anxiety associated with a new baby is to at least think about what you would like to have happen and make your preferences known to your partner, support system, and your healthcare team. Sometimes it seems like the focus is just on the birth

CHAPTER 2: **The Fourth Trimester**   25

plan (see Chapter 1), but what about after you've had your baby? Do you need a plan? Do you wing it? Do you just get annoyed when things don't go how you imagined? Like when family members show up at your house after the baby is born, hoping to have an impromptu meet and greet.

The word plan is a practical and straightforward term often used in preparing for life after birth and the fourth trimester, but I prefer to frame the conversation to be more about what your wishes are after birth. When I work with families and new moms, I help them articulate their postpartum wishes, which they can use as a guide after their baby is born. The type of things that you may want to consider communicating in your postpartum wish list will include:

1. How do you plan to feed your baby? Breast, bottle, or a combination of the two?

2. How soon after you give birth would you like visitors?

3. Who will be in your postpartum support network? (i.e., family, friends, doula, night nurse)

4. Will you prepare meals in advance and freeze them? Or decide to order take out, have a meal train set-up, or get help from your partner, family, or friends?

5. Will you have someone designated to help you and your baby get to your check-ups and doctor's visits?

6. How will you and your partner split household responsibilities so that you can heal and focus on caring for yourself and your new baby?

7. Have you planned to talk with your employer about when you will return from maternity leave? Will you be staying at home with your baby?

8. What household supplies, personal toiletries will you need to buy in preparation? (i.e., Sanitary pads, toilet tissue, paper towels, laundry detergent, soap). Will someone shop for you? Will you shop online?

Postpartum Life

What to Expect

The days and weeks after you have your baby are beautiful and exciting but can also be one of the most vulnerable times for you as a new mom. You've probably heard people say be sure to take care of yourself, but that's not always an easy task when your body is recovering from birth. You're exhausted and just trying to figure out how to adjust to the new normal of motherhood. After giving birth, the important thing to be aware of is being in tune with how you're feeling physically and emotionally. Making sure that you eat nutritiously balanced meals, sleep (when you can – which is usually easiest when your baby sleeps), and accepting help from your village (or making plans to find one – hint, hint cue the postpartum wish list).

Another thing to note is that you will most likely see your doctor or midwife at around 6 to 8 weeks after you have your baby, but it is recognized that this may not be soon enough for some moms. So it is crucial to reach out to your healthcare providers with questions and concerns in the interim. The American College of Obstetricians and Gynecologists (ACOG) recommends that a check-in occurs either in person or by phone in the first few weeks after giving birth to ensure that moms and babies are not experiencing major postpartum issues that would require immediate attention. [2] Unfortunately, some insurance companies may not have jumped on this bandwagon, making reimbursement a challenge.

Next, I'll talk about some signs and symptoms that may indicate that you should reach out to your healthcare provider for further medical advice or treatment. It's also important that your partner or support person(s) be aware of what to look out for as well, since they may be the first person to notice a change in you.

Warning Signs

Now that we've covered some of the basic things that you should know before welcoming your bundle of joy, let's talk about potential signs indicating something may not be right. You and your partner should be on the lookout for the following:

- Are you in any unexplained pain?
- Do you suddenly have unexplained headaches?
- Do you have a fever?
- Are you dizzy or lightheaded?

- Is the rate at which you're bleeding abnormal? – as in soaking a large sanitary pad within an hour or less?
- Do you feel like you cannot complete tasks like showering or bathing without help?
- Do you notice any swelling near your vagina or at your incision site if you had a c-section?

The questions above are basic thoughts to consider in screening for post-birth warning signs and are not meant to substitute for the advice or care that you receive from your healthcare provider. In some cases, your situation could be considered a medical emergency that requires a 911 call. Whenever in doubt, seek medical attention.

For a more comprehensive list, the Association of Women's Health, Obstetric, and Neonatal Nurses (AWHONN) has developed a helpful checklist that I recommend you keep handy. You can find it on the resources list on my website at *www.MercedesThomas.com*.

Hormonal & Emotional Changes
Postpartum Hair Loss

Hair thinning and hair loss are two frightening truths in the postpartum period that many women experience two to four months after giving birth. It can range from increased shedding of hair strands while combing your hair to your hair falling out in clumps. Honestly, this is a regular occurrence, even though it can be distressing. I'm here to tell you that in most cases, if you don't have any pre-existing conditions (like thyroid imbalances or dietary deficiencies), your luscious hair will get back to what it used to be or close to it. That may take some time, though, even as much as a year. I know you're probably wondering if there is anything you can do about postpartum hair loss. Although there isn't a one size fits all solution, research shows that in some women, supplementation with iron and biotin can be effective in strengthening hair and preventing excessive hair loss. [3]

Emotional & Mental Health

As a new mom, your feelings and emotions can be all over the place, much like when you were pregnant. This is totally expected and normal. Your emotions could range from crying to even feeling a little sad or blue.

This brings me to the baby blues, which according to the American Pregnancy Association, is experienced by 70 to 80% of new mothers. It can include mood swings, sadness, exhaustion, uncontrollable crying, and difficulty sleeping (unrelated to the baby). The important thing to note is that the "baby blues" usually subsides within two weeks after giving birth, which is one of the differentiating factors from postpartum depression. [4]

Postpartum depression (PPD) is a critical topic of discussion. It's more common than most people realize, affecting 1 in 8 women. [5] To put that in perspective, for every 8 women you walk past on any given day, let's say in a grocery store or shopping mall, one of them will have been diagnosed with PPD. PPD is characterized by feelings of anger, scary thoughts – like wanting to harm your baby, not feeling competent in caring for your baby, and even isolating yourself from your partner and loved ones. Furthermore, PPD can be more common in women who have a history of depression, poverty, experienced preterm birth, had infertility issues, and have experienced stressful or traumatic life events. [5]

Since there are many different facets of postpartum mental health to be considered and treatment requires individualized and specialized care, it must be said that PPD falls under the perinatal mood and anxiety disorders (PMADS) umbrella. This encompasses many mood-related diagnoses that affect new mothers and includes anxiety, obsessive-compulsive disorder (OCD), post-traumatic stress disorder (PTSD), bipolar disorder, and postpartum psychosis. [6]

Now that we've done a quick overview of postpartum mental health disorders, I want to make something clear. If you or anyone you know is struggling to control their emotions or having scary thoughts, one, you're not alone, and two, you're still a good mother! It's also imperative for you to know that should you feel "off" in any way or have those very frightening or troubling thoughts that you should seek help. Please know that there is nothing to be ashamed of for doing so. You can seek help from many places, including a mental health professional like a therapist, psychiatrist, or a nurse practitioner specifically trained to care for psychiatric

CHAPTER 2: **The Fourth Trimester** 31

clients. Depending on the type of therapy or treatment needed, you may even be able to establish care virtually. If you don't know where to start, it's a good idea to reach out to your OB-GYN or midwife for a referral to a local mental health professional. Also, you can find a list of mental health resources in Appendix A.

I created the Mommy Mood Tracker™ for you to use as a means to "check-in" with yourself and monitor how you're feeling in the early days and weeks after the birth of your baby. If you start to see a trend of sad and stressed days, please check in with your partner or a trusted support person and your healthcare provider. You can download the pdf version at *www.MercedesThomas.com/resources.*

MOMMY MOOD TRACKER™

WEEK ___

+THIS TRACKER IS FOR INFORMATIONAL PURPOSES ONLY AND DOES NOT REPLACE THE GUIDANCE AND CARE OF YOUR PRIMARY CARE OR MENTAL HEALTH PROVIDER.

MONDAY	TUESDAY	WEDNESDAY	THURSDAY
FRIDAY	SATURDAY	SUNDAY	

KEY:
- 😐 FEELING, BLAH BUT OKAY
- 🙂 HAPPY & CONTENT
- 🙁 FEELING SAD & I'M NOT OKAY
- ☹️ FEELING STRESSED & OVERWHELMED

© 2020 MERCEDES THOMAS, ALL RIGHTS RESERVED.

CHAPTER 3

Baby Care & Tips

*"They eat, they crap, they sleep.
And if they're crying, they need to do one of the three,
and they're having trouble doing it. Real simple."*

—Matthew McConaughey

Next up, let's meet Jennifer, a mother who just had her baby Liam around five days before we met. Baby Liam was born at a baby-friendly hospital. Simply put, this is a hospital where the staff is trained to support you in meeting your breastfeeding goals. Also, hospitals with this designation don't offer breast milk substitutes (like formula) unless there is a medically indicated reason. I met Jennifer at her home to help her with baby Liam's latch, which caused her incredible pain while breastfeeding him. Thankfully the pain was short-lived. With my guidance and much determination on her part (this is always a huge part of the breastfeeding puzzle), Jennifer was able to tweak baby Liam's positioning at the breast to get a deeper latch. Eventually, he was able to breastfeed like a champ.

A week later, during our follow-up appointment, Jennifer reported that baby Liam was waking up every 1 ½ to 2 hours to breastfeed, was having at least 6 to 8 wet diapers every twenty-four hours, and was pooping around 3 to 4 times per day. I was so pleased to hear that Jennifer and her husband, Mike, were settling into their new lives as parents.

So now, back to you and your baby. Now that you've given birth, how in the world are you supposed to care for this tiny little human, you ask?!? All of the excitement, emotions, and fear (yes, fear) have set in, and you're now responsible for this tiny, little baby. I'm here to tell you not to worry because I'm going to keep it simple.

So here goes the big secret that you should know before we begin. The three basic needs of a baby are to eat, sleep, and poop (ESP)! Repeat it with me: eat, sleep, and poop. So, when all else fails to go as planned because honestly, there's virtually no way to have a rigid parenting plan as a new mom of a newborn, keep the ESP mantra in your mind to recenter yourself. Most importantly, if you remember nothing else on your most exhausting day, remember to remain as flexible as possible.

The Nitty Gritty on Pooping and Peeing

Pooping and Peeing aka "The Elimination"
Like baby Liam, most healthy newborns will have 6 to 8 wet diapers per day, but I want to backtrack to the "first poop" babies have after they're born, known as meconium stool. Meconium is thick, sticky, and dark green – almost looks

black in color and is hard to clean, but we'll talk about diapering in the next section. After meconium comes the transitional stool around day 2 or 3 of life, which is usually a greenish-brown to greenish-yellow color and is thinner and less sticky.

Breastfed babies' poop usually has a very characteristic mustard yellow color, which often looks "seedy," and many parents nervously think that their baby has diarrhea, but the thin consistency is expected. Many breastfed babies may stool from as little as twice per day to as much as after every single feeding. Now, how's that for elimination?

Formula-fed babies' poop typically ranges from a yellowish tan color to brown. It is also usually more firm. However, firm shouldn't be confused for hard, which can be a sign that your baby is constipated. Generally, formula fed babies don't poop as frequently as breastfed babies. On average, you can expect them to poop on a daily basis or even skip a day or two.

I talked about normal pooping and urinating patterns, but what should you keep an eye out for? The list below includes some of the things that may be worth calling your baby's healthcare provider about.

- Mucous in the poop (think runny nose).
- Streaks of blood in your baby's poop.
- No poop for more than 2 – 3 days in a row.
- Stools that are hard and resemble small pebbles.

- Your baby draws his or her legs up toward their stomach, in pain, while attempting to poop.
- If by day 4 of life, you notice that you're changing less than 6 diapers in a 24 hour period.

Diapering Your Baby

Maybe you've changed zero diapers or hundreds, but spoiler alert, I'm going to go through the basics here for mamas who need the down and dirty of diapering – pun intended.

First, let's start with some sweet truths, like the act of changing your baby's diaper can be a great moment for a new mama and baby to bond. There's an opportunity to get face to face with your baby, make eye contact, and time to talk with him or her and wait for those cute little coos and smiles in response. Your baby is never too young for you to start talking to them, not to mention this is a great way to start building on language development from an early age.

Diapering Rules to Live By

The first rule of diapering is to have all of the essentials near the diaper changing table or area. This includes diapers, wipes, diaper cream, or petroleum jelly. Although they're optional, creams offer an additional layer of protection from stool and urine, which due to acidity, can sometimes irritate your baby's bottom.

Of all of the rules, the most important two are never leaving your baby unaccompanied on the changing table and always keeping one hand on him or her as an additional safety measure to prevent an accidental fall.

The Diaper Changing Strategy

You'll want to start by undoing the tabs on the diaper and laying it flat on the changing table. Next, lift your baby's legs up gently and place the clean diaper underneath the dirty diaper you plan to change. Just leave it there for the time being. This trick allows for an extra barrier and serves as a way to protect yourself, which I'll talk about in a second.

Next, brace yourself and undo the tabs on the dirty diaper. If your baby has pooped, I suggest wiping the excess poop off with the dirty diaper's unsoiled portion (if there is a "clean" area). Then, fold the dirty diaper clean side up underneath your baby. Keeping the dirty diaper folded under your baby is a way to protect the clean diaper underneath and offer an extra protective layer.

Up next is using wipes to gently but thoroughly clean your baby's genital area from front to back. This is especially important if you have a baby girl and to avoid introducing bacteria into her vaginal area. After you're done wiping the genital area, you can apply your diaper cream. I recommend one with zinc in the ingredients due to its skin protectant properties. Finally, if you have a baby boy, something to keep in mind, unless you like being sprayed (insert smiles), is being prepared to cover his penis. This can be done with the flap of the clean diaper which you already have placed underneath him.

Bathing Your Baby

Giving a bath is another vital skill to have as a new parent. For many families, the first bath is considered a rite of passage for babies and one for the books – the baby memory book. Two things to note are:

1. If your baby's umbilical cord stump is still attached, you'll want to keep that area as dry as possible until it falls off.

2. If your baby boy has been circumcised, your pediatrician may recommend that you hold off on the bath until the penis has healed.

Once you're home, it'll be time for the first sponge bath on your own. But do not worry, soon you'll be a pro.

As with changing the diaper, you'll want to gather all of your supplies. I recommend a gentle, unscented cleanser, a washcloth, 2 towels, a soft hairbrush, and a clean, dry outfit. If you have a safe, clean area near your kitchen or bathroom sink, many parents prefer this area for close proximity to a water source. You can graduate to a baby bathtub once the umbilical cord has completely fallen off and your baby is big enough to do so safely. Remember, you don't have to bathe your new baby every day. You can skip a day in between because, let's face it, a brand spanking new baby isn't "dirty."

CHAPTER 3: **Baby Care & Tips** 39

These are the steps:

- Ensure the room where you're bathing the baby is warm and free of cold drafts.
- Fill your sink or basin, whichever you choose, with lukewarm water.
- Lay down 1 clean towel on the flat, clean surface of your choice (set the second to the side, you'll use it later)
- Undress your baby and place him or her onto the clean towel and use the second clean towel to cover those parts that aren't being washed.
- Wash gently with a washcloth from the cleanest area, which would be the face ending with feet and genital area (remember to avoid the umbilical button area until it's dried, but you may gently clean around the outside of it).
- After washing the face with plain water, you may opt to add a small quarter-sized amount of gentle cleanser to the water versus adding it directly to the washcloth. This helps to minimize the drying effect that soap can have on the skin.
- When cleaning the genital area, be sure to gently clean from front to back for baby girls. For boys, remember to gently cleanse the penis, and if circumcised, follow the recommendations of the licensed healthcare provider who performed the procedure until the penis has healed.
- Finally, wrap your baby in a dry clean towel.

Newborn Appearance

Peeling Skin

It's normal for your new baby's skin to look as though it's peeling; in fact, many full-term healthy babies appear this way, so there's usually no need to worry or to pull out any special exfoliating tools. After all, your baby has their whole adult life ahead of them to use those. An unscented lotion is okay to use after bathing.

Umbilical Cord Stump

We've talked a little about umbilical cord stumps already, but as a summary, you'll want to avoid submerging your baby into the water for a bath and just stick with a sponge bath until the cord stump has completely dried. A week or two after it's dried, you can expect the stump to fall off, revealing just the belly button.

Always remember that if you notice any discharge, oozing, or odor coming from the umbilical cord to contact your child's healthcare provider right away as this could be a sign of infection. You'll also want to refer to your child's doctor if you notice any bulging around or near the belly button because this could indicate that he or she has an umbilical hernia. Not to worry, most umbilical hernias are harmless and pretty common in babies.

Sleeping Patterns

Oh, sleep, that five-letter word that so many parents seem to be desperately researching. Parents are hoping to crack the "sleep code" to learn all of the coveted secrets so that they can help their baby to sleep through the night. Well, I'm here to tell you that newborn babies sleep an average of 16 to 17 hours a day. However, that is not 16 to 17 consecutive hours of sleep and may only last for up to 2 hours at a time. So, believe me when I say it's normal for your new baby to not be sleeping through the night and that biologically they're supposed to be waking to eat. You will eventually get your new bundle of joy on a schedule, but the newborn period is best spent bonding, getting to know your baby, and letting them eat, sleep, and poop when they can and need to. You can read more on sleep in Chapter 8.

Swaddling Your Baby

Swaddling is a magical skill to have, and even better, it's oh so simple once you've learned it. If you think about the fact that your baby has spent nine months being carried by you, then it all makes sense.

Swaddling offers a sense of security, boundaries, and warmth, simulating the safe environment that they grew to love leading up to their birth. The thing about swaddling is that although it helps babies calm down, it really should not serve as a substitute for your gentle touch or to keep your baby sleeping for hours because, as mentioned before, they should be waking to eat in those early weeks.

One trick is to swaddle but leave your baby's arms free to come up to the natural resting position, which is often near their face. Freeing those little hands will also allow you to notice one of the early feeding cues, like bringing hands to the mouth. I'll talk more about this in Chapter 5.

Things That Seem Scary, But Are Pretty Common

Witch's Milk

The term "witch's milk" sounds super scary, and no, it has nothing to do with a witch whatsoever. Witch's milk can be alarming when parents notice it but simply put, it is milk that is secreted from the breasts of babies and can be seen in baby girls and boys. Without getting too technical, the secretion of the milk is related to maternal hormones, and there is no need for concern because it's normal.

What In The Discharge?!?

Another concerning but normal finding in newborn baby girls is a blood-tinged mucus-like discharge that comes from the vagina, which is also linked to maternal hormones and will eventually stop.

Newborn Rash

Does it itch? Will it ever go away? Does it hurt? What can I do to treat it? These are all questions I've received over the last decade from parents regarding their newborn baby's skin. In fact, dermatology is one of my favorite topics. The truth is, many times, I get to tell parents that the majority of rashes in children don't lead to scary endings.

Anyway, back to the infamous newborn rash, which is usually concentrated on the face. It appears as bumps or pimples with reddened patches (this can be seen easier on fair skin babies) mixed in with the occasional peeling of the skin. Although the rash looks pretty bad sometimes, it's normal and also a result of those pesky maternal hormones passed from mother to baby. No treatment is needed. Heat and scented skin products can make the rash worse, so as previously recommended, try to stick with unscented mild and gentle cleansers and lotions.

CHAPTER 4

Adapting to Motherhood

"The biggest thing I remember is that there was just no transition. You hit the ground, diapering."

—Paul Reiser

The setting for this story goes way back to my undergraduate college days. Shout out to the Nell Hodgson Woodruff School of Nursing in Atlanta, GA. Now that's a mouthful of a name for you, isn't it?

Anyway, one day, a group of my classmates and I were talking about parenthood. Some of my classmates were already knee-deep into parenting, whereas motherhood for me at the time was something I knew I wanted but was not anywhere in the five-year plan, if you know what I mean. I recall saying I wanted to wait until I was married and "ready" to have my first child. One of my classmates interjected and said that you can never truly prepare to be a parent and that there was no perfect time to do so. When she said this, I'll admit I kind of blew the statement off since it didn't make any sense to me at the time. I'm the planner of all planners and live my life as such, so that's exactly how I would follow the path to motherhood.

Well, here comes another spoiler alert; it turns out she was right! Imagine not being able to plan every aspect of having your first child. I believe that you can be prepared, but being ready for anything that can and will happen is just not possible, and I learned this first hand when my time came.

Adapting to motherhood is a mother, pun intended! As I like to say, "it's a crazy, beautiful, tiring state of managing to be a superhero while sacrificing it all for your child(ren)." So now that you've researched everything that you could think of when it comes to babies, googling, tirelessly reading all the blogs you can find, polling all the mom groups, and reading books, now what?

The truth is, I wish I could tell you just what motherhood would be like. But since it's such an individualized experience like no other, there is no one size fits all answer.

Think about this scenario: your friend (mom A), who has had five pregnancies, is literally in love with the act of being pregnant. She never experienced a pregnancy-associated ache or pain, and get this, she never experienced morning sickness one time! Like really, who is this woman? Then you have mom B, a first-time mother who can't even look at food without feeling nauseous. She's sure that she has every pregnancy ailment in the book. As her bundle of joy is growing, she describes the feeling that her "ribs are being rearranged daily." Not to mention, after her fourth pregnancy pillow, she is convinced she will never get another good night's sleep again.

See how this works? Two different women experienced pregnancy in entirely different ways, which may shape their perceptions and memories related to pregnancy.

In this chapter, I want to give you some tools to help you find your way along the path to transitioning to motherhood. I'll share some of my must-have products, suggestions on finding balance, and tips on how to take care of yourself, aka self-care.

The Nitty Gritty on Adapting to Motherhood

Time to cue the bucket list. Believe it or not, I don't really have one outside of a list of places I want to travel to. For me, vacation and travel are life, but that doesn't mean that I don't keep mental notes of things that I'd like to do or accomplish during my time here on earth.

Transitioning into motherhood shouldn't have to be the death of the old you, but more like a fusion of who you were before having a child coupled with new life experiences, constant learning, and adapting. My suggestion is to think of some of the things you would like to experience or do and develop a flexible plan for making them happen. For instance, you can still travel, and you should, but you may need to adapt how often you travel or your transportation mode to get to your destination.

Finding Your Village

If you take anything away from this chapter, please take this piece of advice because you will need it. Finding a village is essential as a mother and can be life-changing for you, your baby, and your partner.

Self-care Is So Important

Self-care, you literally can't go anywhere or read anything without seeing this word somewhere as it pertains to so many aspects of life, honestly. It's an overused catchphrase that means you should set aside time to take care of yourself. Yes, you need to take care of yourself because there's only one of you.

As mothers, we give so much to so many, and of course, you want to give your time, heart, and soul to your baby and family, but you have to ensure that your mind, body, and emotions are intact to do so.

Self-care comes in so many different forms. It can be napping when your baby rests because sleep is even more essential and hard to come by when you're a new parent. Self-care can be taking a walk or going out for a jog or run. Endorphins are produced within your body while exercising, and that can help kick stress to the curb. Now keep on reading for a list of self-care ideas.

Self-care Checklist:

- Eat a healthy meal – think lean protein, veggies, and whole grains
- Take a social media break – you can just log out or take it a step further and delete the app off of your phone
- Spend 15 to 30 minutes reading a book or magazine
- Get outside and enjoy some fresh air and sunshine
- Go for a walk or jog
- Take time out to do absolutely nothing
- Netflix and chill
- Listen to your favorite music
- Get a manicure, pedicure, or both! – if you don't have the time to get to a nail salon, do it yourself (DIY) at home. Even if you're not the most creative person, there are so many options, like adhesive nail polish strips. I have to say the brand that I tried survived all the excessive hand washing I do at work and hand sanitizer that I use.
- Meditate
- Journal
- Do some yoga or just stretch
- Eat one of your favorite foods
- Light a candle and put your feet up – think aromatherapy

- Take a "cat nap" – I've never had a cat, and they're certainly not my favorite pet, but my mom always says this, and it's just an expression for taking a quick nap. A great time to do this is when your partner is home or when your baby is sleeping.
- Take a bubble bath

Finding Your New Normal

Once your baby is here, what will life look like? Well, the answer to that is we don't always know as mothers. The key is to try your best to be flexible and adapt when needed. In being flexible, think about how you can weave in the pieces of your life that are most important to you and will keep you sane. Yes, I said the "s" word, sane. Part of finding your new normal is having an outlet to be you so that you still have an identity outside of being a mom. Keep in mind that this doesn't mean that your little one isn't your primary focus, especially in the early years.

One way to maintain your sanity is to be very intentional and realistic about the goals you plan to set, pursue, and achieve. Think of where you see your life going and aim to take steps to move in that direction. While working towards your goals, try your best to set limits on things and people, if needed. Last but not least, give yourself grace and the freedom to adjust your pace if needed.

Another consideration is to think about new routines that will accommodate your physical and mental well-being.

This is one way to ensure that you're able to be present and whole for your new baby and family. Examples include regular exercise, talking with a therapist, or even venting to a trusted and supportive friend. Try taking time to recharge by using one of the suggestions mentioned in the self-care checklist above.

You'll also want to think about ways to keep your other relationships going, like the one with your partner, friends, and family, because staying connected is so important. In the early days, I know how hard it can be to do anything outside of focusing on your baby but starting with at least 10 intentional minutes of connecting with your partner by discussing your day is essential. The icing on the cake is if you're able to sit down to have dinner together while you discuss. My advice is to do what you can, even if you start small initially, and adapt as needed.

Returning to Work

If you plan to return to work in some capacity, there will be a new routine for you and your baby to adjust to. One of the best ways to tackle your return and make it less stressful is to prepare. Preparing can be done in many ways.

One of the first steps is to figure out what your financial responsibilities are. Many new moms find that they may want to return but work fewer hours in the beginning and slowly increase back to full-time. Or maybe you just plan on cutting back your hours indefinitely. You'll want to run the numbers to see if it's doable.

Once you determine your work status, you'll want to discuss this with your employer and fill out any necessary paperwork that human resources may require relating to your return after maternity leave and employer sponsored benefits. You will also want to discuss plans like pumping at work, and we'll talk more about this in Chapter 5.

Next, you'll want to figure out child care for your new baby. Decisions like if you'll use daycare, a nanny, or a babysitter will be necessary. If you're using a childcare provider outside of your home, factoring that stop into your morning and evening commute will need to be a consideration. Once you figure out your childcare plan, I highly suggest you do a couple of practice runs of your drive to work and your child's care provider. Doing so will allow you to estimate the amount of time you can expect to commute each day.

Another helpful step in preparing for your return to work is the act of getting everything ready, or as much as you possibly can, the night before. This will eliminate scrambling around in the morning to find stuff and keep you on schedule.

Last but not least, is my favorite hack and a fantastic "trick" to ease into going back to work. I was lucky enough to have this happen naturally, but you may be able to make it work for you too. If possible, try to return to work on a Friday or towards the end of your workweek if you have a non-traditional Monday through Friday work schedule. One reason is, you'll be missing your baby and dealing with all the

CHAPTER 4: **Adapting to Motherhood** 53

emotions that may come with that, plus figuring out a whole new routine. So, starting back towards the end of the week will allow you the weekend or whatever your off days are to tweak your routine and see what worked for you and baby and prepare for the next week accordingly.

CHAPTER 5

Breastfeeding & Bottle Feeding

"Nurturing and nourishing your baby are two of the greatest joys of motherhood, and one day you'll look back and wonder why you ever worried about doing either one the wrong way."

—MERCEDES THOMAS, CPNP, IBCLC

By now, there's no surprise that I'm a breastfeeding advocate and a certified lactation consultant. But as a pediatric nurse practitioner, it's my responsibility to support parents to safely feed their babies whether they choose breast milk or formula, and this chapter will give you the nitty-gritty on both.

Before we talk about the specifics, I want to give you an overview. In Chapter 3, I mentioned the "ESP" (eat, sleep, poop) cycle that babies should be following to grow and thrive. The eating part of the cycle should lead to steady weight gain, and although many newborn babies lose up to 10% of their birth weight, in pediatric land, we expect babies to regain their birth weight by two weeks of age.

After the two-week milestone is met, it is expected for most babies to gain around one ounce per day. Your child's healthcare provider will track weight gain on a growth chart, which gives percentiles to serve as a benchmark for how well your baby is growing in length, height, and head circumference.

Keep in mind that formula and breastfed babies grow at different rates. It is preferred that healthy breastfed babies have their weight and growth tracked on the World Health Organization (WHO) growth charts versus the standard CDC growth charts, which are more representative of babies who are primarily formula-fed.

The Nitty Gritty on Infant Feeding

The Newborn Stomach

Let's start off with the average size of the newborn stomach. On day one, your baby's tummy is similar to the size of a marble; on day three, the size of a ping pong ball, and on day 10, the size of an egg. See below for a visual along with the typical amount of milk that a newborn baby's stomach can hold.

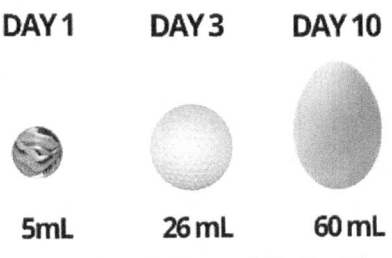

DAY 1	DAY 3	DAY 10
5 mL	26 mL	60 mL

© 2020 Mercedes Thomas, All Rights Reserved.

CHAPTER 5: **Breastfeeding & Bottle Feeding** 57

Hunger Cues

I bet you're wondering how on earth you're supposed to know when your baby is hungry. I mean, it's not like he or she can talk! The good news is that there are some pretty common signs that babies give us when they're ready to eat. The signs range from very subtle and cute to angry and loud. The key here is to avoid letting your baby get to the irritated and loud phase of hunger. If your baby gets to what I refer to as the "point of no return," also known as the angry and loud phase, you will want to start by trying your best to comfort him or her to allow a little time to settle down.

Cute and subtle hunger signs or those that happen early on are:
- Rooting – the act of moving the head from side to side in reaction to touching the cheeks or lips
- Tongue thrusting
- Opening of mouth

The irritated and loud hunger signs or those that are hailed as late signs include:
- Crying
- Grimacing
- Uncontrollable flailing

What to Expect In the Early Days
The first few days of life for a newborn are literally full of the mantra ESP! In terms of eating, you should expect your baby to be pretty alert in the first 1-2 hours after delivery,

but sleep quite a bit after that. So you'll want to maximize that period right after delivery and any time after to get in as much skin-to-skin as possible. Skin-to-skin will allow your baby to not only be close to you but have access to the breast if you decide to nurse your baby.

On day two, you should expect a more alert baby, and his or her hunger cues should begin to be more noticeable to you. By day 2 or 3, you can also expect the infamous "cluster feeding" that occurs in newborns and sometimes makes a startling encore if you decide to breastfeed into the toddler years. Trust me, I know from personal experience. Anyway, back to cluster feeding, which is a period of time when your baby seems to continuously or frequently feed. This can last for hours, and when I say hours, I really mean it! When this time comes, and it will come, I recommend riding it out by keeping your baby close and selecting a baby-friendly self-care activity from the list in Chapter 4, like taking time to "Netflix and chill." Finally, as a rule of thumb, you should expect to feed your newborn 8 to 12 times per day.

Breastfeeding Basics
Exclusive Breastfeeding
The act of exclusive breastfeeding is deciding to only feed your baby breast milk without formula supplementation. This is a goal that many moms strive for, and it's definitely doable with the proper support. Although it's sometimes

effortless for many breastfeeding parents, there's also the potential for the most natural act of feeding your baby, to begin with, some challenges.

Hopefully, by the time your baby is born, you've taken a prenatal breastfeeding course, as suggested in Chapter 1, but if not, there's still time. I strongly recommend expectant parents take a breastfeeding class before having their baby. You can usually find prenatal breastfeeding classes at your local hospital or through recommendations from a community-based breastfeeding group like La Leche League. You can also try searching for IBCLC's who may be offering them in-person or virtually. I offer a virtual course to teach parents the information needed to prepare for their breastfeeding journey from the comfort of their own home. More information can be found on my website at *www.MercedesThomas.com.*

The Basics of Exclusive Breastfeeding

Your exclusive breastfeeding journey begins after you give birth, and you can get off to a great start by doing skin to skin. You might be saying to yourself by now that skin-to-skin seems to be important, and you would be very correct! Early on in the first hour after you give birth, you may be able to observe the magical "breast crawl" where your little one will find his or her way to your breast by merely using his or her legs and arms to move around on your chest. Smell and sight are some of the primary reflexes present in babies early on, like rooting, which helps them to find your breast.

During the hours and first couple of days after you give birth, your body will produce colostrum. Although it may be thin in appearance and small in amount, it is breast milk and packed with nutrients. It's the perfect first "food" that your baby needs.

You may also consider gently expressing some colostrum from your breasts. This can be done with gentle massaging of your breasts, stroking backward and then forward with one hand, to help get your baby interested in latching on to your breast in the beginning. The great thing about colostrum is that it will help stabilize your baby's blood sugar and help get the ESP cycle going with a heavy emphasis on the "P." Pooping is very important for new babies and allows their bodies to start getting rid of meconium, which is a good sign that your baby is getting enough milk.

How to Get Started with Breastfeeding

One of the fundamental but central aspects of breastfeeding is the latch that you've most likely heard about. Will it be all you dreamed of, effortless or magical? In my humble opinion, the act of initiating your breastfeeding relationship is magical all in itself. However, answering how easy latching your baby will be can depend on several factors. Breastfeeding does take some work and preparation and may not be the most natural of acts for your baby.

I can tell you that if you know the basics of a good latch and positioning your baby, you are far more likely to get off to a good start with breastfeeding, and that is my hope for you because knowledge is truly empowering.

The Nitty Gritty on Latching

So far, we've talked a lot about the benefits of skin-to-skin and how it can help to get breastfeeding off to a great start. While you're doing skin-to-skin, it is a great time to start working on latching your baby to the breast.

Here are four basic steps to follow:

1. Align your baby's chest to your stomach and line his or her nose up with your nipple.

2. Take your hand and shape it as if you were about to grasp a large hamburger. If you're not a burger fan, think of shaping your hand into a "c" shape and flip your hand so that your fingers are facing down and place your hand around your breast to support and gently lift it. Check to make sure your fingers are not directly on top of your areola and that there is about an inch of skin showing between your areola and fingers.

3. Support the back of your baby's head with your other arm and hand. Gently stroke your baby's top lip with your nipple, pausing at the lower lip to allow your baby to open his or her mouth widely. Be patient with this step and let the baby be the boss and lead.

4. Once your baby's mouth is opened wide and the head is slightly tilted back, aim your nipple towards the roof of the mouth, letting the chin be the first point of contact with your breast. Then guide your baby so that the majority of your areola is inside of his or her mouth.

How Do You Know the Latch Is Good?

Before getting to the list of tips to make sure your baby has a good latch, I want to start by saying that breastfeeding is not meant to be, nor should it be painful. However, there may be some discomfort associated with breastfeeding in the beginning because it's a new skill for you and your baby to learn and may take some trial and error (which is perfectly okay) to get it right. Having said that, if breastfeeding is ever painful, even after trying different positions, unlatching your baby, and readjusting the latch, then you should strongly consider reaching out to a lactation professional for help.

Here are some signs that I'd like to share with you that let you know that your baby is attached to your breast well and is getting enough milk:

1. Your baby's lips are flipped outward.

2. Your baby doesn't have a shallow attachment to your breast, meaning that your nipple and more of the bottom of your areola are inside of his or her mouth than the top portion.

3. Your baby is gaining at least 1 ounce per day.

4. Your baby has numerous wet diapers (at least 6-8) and around 2-3 poopy diapers each day.

5. You can actively hear your baby swallowing your milk.

6. Your baby's jaw moves in a long rhythmic motion.

7. You're not feeling any pain. Remember, discomfort in the first week or so is not out of the ordinary.

CHAPTER 5: **Breastfeeding & Bottle Feeding**   63

8. When your baby is done breastfeeding, your nipple should still appear rounded and not be flattened or creased. If you wear lipstick, envision the shape of the tip of your favorite shade. This would be an example of what your nipple shouldn't look like after your baby is done feeding at the breast.

BREASTFEEDING POSITIONS

How to hold and support your baby

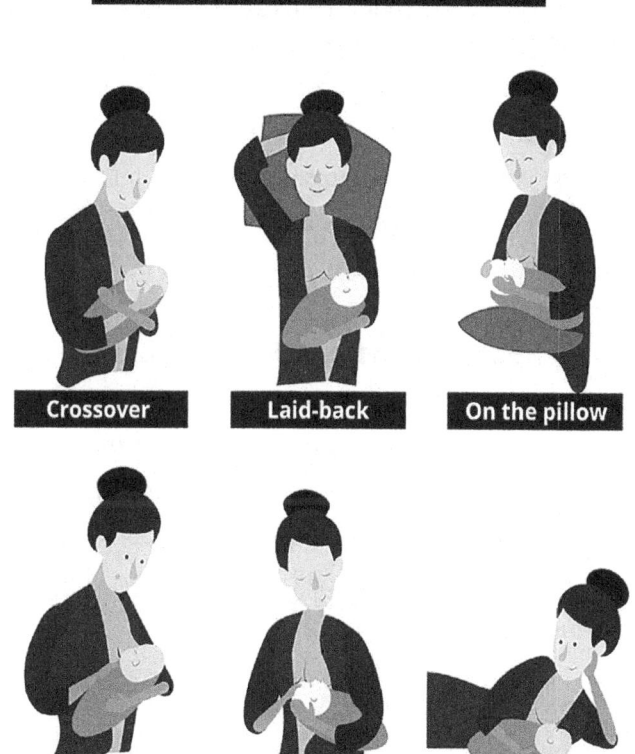

Crossover

Laid-back

On the pillow

Cradle

Football Hold

Side-lying

How Long Should You Breastfeed?

The American Academy of Pediatrics (AAP) recommends that lactating parents exclusively breastfeed for at least six months. Followed by continued breastfeeding, as age-appropriate solid foods are introduced, with the continuation of breastfeeding for one year or longer, if the parent desires and the baby is still interested. [7]

Additionally, the World Health Organization (WHO) recommends that babies be exclusively breastfed and not receive any other foods or liquids until six months of age, and continuing to breastfeed for up to two years or longer. [8]

As you can see, it is strongly recommended that you breastfeed your infant. And that you continue to do so for as long as you and your baby want to continue. This timeframe can range from birth through toddlerhood, depending on your personal breastfeeding goals.

Tips to Boost and Maintain Your Supply

One of the most common questions that I get from the breastfeeding clients I work with and teach is how to increase their breast milk supply. So, I'm going to share some of my top tips to combat low milk supply. Before I do, I'd like to add that there is no magic wand to wave when it comes to your breast milk supply.

There are cookies, brownies, teas, and concoctions sold by many companies selling a promise that the product most likely cannot live up to, which is a massive boost in your breast milk supply. Then there are electrolyte drinks, which many women swear by to increase their breast milk supply. Now what I will say is that there's no evidence-based research that currently proves this theory. What is possible is that a dehydrated mom does feel like she's having an increase in supply because she is now better hydrated. So again, is this a magical phenomenon? No, but it is a natural reaction that can occur in the body when hydrated.

On the complete opposite end of the spectrum are mothers who may have hormone imbalances, medical conditions, or a history of surgical breast procedures that may limit their ability to naturally produce an adequate supply needed to exclusively breastfeed their baby.

I would strongly suggest that moms with a known medical history that could become a barrier to achieving their breastfeeding goals find a lactation professional. For example, breast surgery or known hormone imbalances would be common reasons to seek out advice. A knowledgeable International Board Certified Lactation Consultant (IBCLC) and your healthcare provider would be two professionals to consult with prenatally. Some ways to find a local IBCLC referral include asking your child's pediatrician, your obstetrician, midwife, or even through a reputable breastfeeding support group like La Leche League or a local WIC office.

Another option is to search for an IBCLC local to you using the directory on ilca.org. Honestly, you don't have to wait until you have a breastfeeding issue to see a lactation consultant.

Many insurance companies will cover these visits, which is an excellent resource for any mom who is new to breastfeeding.

Now back to the breast milk supply tips that I wanted to share with you (see Appendix A):

- **Let the MILK FLOW:** Yes, you read that right! Breastfeed that baby. It doesn't matter how many times (cue the cluster feeding). Hand express, or whip out that hospital-grade pump. The method doesn't matter as long as your baby is getting that liquid gold. Choose one of these or a combination of them and repeat every 2 to 3 hours. Power pumping is also a great way to rev up your milk production.

- **Warmth:** A rice sock (inexpensive and easy to make), warmed gel packs, a warm washcloth, or a steamy warm shower all do the trick to soften your breasts and combat those awful clogs and maximize production. Apply warmth before breastfeeding or pumping.

- **Massage "the girls":** We could all use a spa day, especially us mamas! But for now, let's settle for a breast massage. Start with the gentle massage of your breasts and some kneading (always gentle). This helps to stimulate milk, let down. You can also grab one of those handy battery-operated massagers if you'd like to give your hands a rest. My top tip is that sometimes you can find one at your local dollar store.

CHAPTER 5: **Breastfeeding & Bottle Feeding** 67

Feeding Breast Milk from a Bottle

By now, you may be wondering what your options are if you want to give your baby breast milk but don't have the ability or desire to latch him or her to your breast. Some common options are to exclusively pump or feed your baby human milk supplied by a donor.

Exclusive pumping is expressing or removing milk from the breasts regularly from 8 to 12 times per day and feeding that milk to your baby from a bottle. Some women prefer this option versus latching their baby to their breast for a variety of reasons, but this is no small feat, and although doable, I highly recommend that you seek out support to help you along the way.

Donor milk is obtained from another lactating person and can be obtained from a human milk bank. However, donor milk usually comes at a cost that is generally calculated by the ounce and can be out of budget for many parents. Although some mothers prefer to participate in informal milk sharing, there are risks that should be considered. My best advice is to educate yourself and discuss the pros and cons with a lactation professional and your healthcare provider (see Appendix A).

Other options for removing milk from your breast include hand expression, the use of an electric pump, or a manual hand pump. Hand expression is a powerful technique to learn and can be invaluable to you, especially in the early days as you start learning how to breastfeed your baby. Although

I'll briefly explain the steps to hand express below, a video shows a fantastic demonstration of the technique can be found in Appendix A.

Before you begin, please be sure to wash your hands well, including under your fingernails, and follow these steps:

- Ensure you have a clean wide-brimmed container or spoon (for the colostrum) available to collect the milk.
- Gently massage your breast with warm hands to help get the milk flowing.
- Hold the container near your nipple with one hand and place your opposite hand you're your breast, around 1 to 2 inches away from your nipple, using the upside-down "c" shape hold described earlier in this chapter.
- With firm but gentle pressure, press your fingers and thumb back towards your chest.
- Squeeze gently in a downward motion to express the milk into a clean container or spoon. Release your breast and repeat.

How Much Breast Milk Should I Feed My Baby from the Bottle?

A breastfed baby's volume intake is very unique. Believe it or not, due to the contents and proportions of nutrients, including fats, breast milk is digested much differently than formula. So the magical question that so many mothers ask

CHAPTER 5: **Breastfeeding & Bottle Feeding**

me, and one that I pondered many days as I prepared to return to work after maternity leave, is "how much milk will my baby need to be fed while he or she is away from me?"

Although many mothers plan to exclusively breastfeed and can do so for as long as they wish, the reality is that many women will need to be away from their baby at some point in time.

The Average Daily Amount

From birth to one month of age, the average amount of breast milk needed per day is approximately 24 ounces. By 6 months old, there is a slight increase of up to 30 ounces per day. [9] Depending on the number of feedings per day, this could be 3 to 4 ounces at a time for a baby who is drinking eight bottles per day. This number is a point of reference, even if you're supplementing with formula. You would just subtract the amount of formula you're feeding each day from the average total based on your baby's age and your child's primary care provider's recommendations.

Keep in mind that the average daily amount of breast milk is only relevant if you will be separated from your baby for 24 hours or more. For many, the average time away will be to go run an errand or to leave for work. In these instances, you can figure that you will need to pump (or hand express) and store approximately 1 to 1 ½ ounces of breast milk per hour that you will be away.

Paced Bottle Feeding

Another aspect that you should be familiar with when learning about feeding your new baby is the suck, swallow, breathe (SSB) pattern that newborns must learn to master. This is the natural coordination of actions and reflexes by which your baby can successfully master drinking from a bottle. So as your baby is learning to SSB, think about how hard it would be for them to drink from a bottle where the flow of the milk is fast flowing instead of coming out at a slower controlled rate, which can be achieved using the paced bottle feeding technique.

At some point, you may have heard or learned that babies who are offered bottles will no longer want to breastfeed. However, the part of the story that isn't always clear is that this is usually less from "nipple confusion" (breast versus bottle nipple) and more of "bottle preference" that many babies are prone to.

Breastfeeding usually allows babies to have a slower flow of milk than from a bottle, and let's face it, most anyone prefers the easiest way possible of doing something, and babies are no different.

Paced bottle feeding is a way to allow your baby the time to coordinate their SSB and digest their food at a more natural pace, giving them the chance to recognize that they're full. Selecting a slow flow nipple is preferable as many of the nipples that come with bottles are a "level one," which may have a hole at the top that allows for the milk to flow much

CHAPTER 5: **Breastfeeding & Bottle Feeding** 71

faster than you would want for a newborn baby. If you're wondering, yes, paced bottle feeding can be done whether you're feeding your baby formula or breast milk.

These are the steps to give paced feeding a shot:

- Sit your baby in your lap in a more upright position (approximately at a 45-degree angle).

- Use the nipple on the bottle to gently stroke your baby's lips to get him or her to open them widely.

- Once the bottle is inside the mouth, keep the bottle horizontal to the lips, at approximately a 90-degree angle, to help control the milk flow. Another reference point is to make sure the nipple is only half full versus completely filled with milk.

- Around every 20 to 30 seconds, tilt the bottle downward (with the nipple still inside of the baby's mouth) to slow down the flow of the milk and give your baby time to have a short break.

- Once the bottle is near half full, burp your baby, switch him or her to face the opposite side, and continue feeding.

Breast Milk (aka human milk) Storage Guidelines:

After you express or pump your breast milk, you'll need to store it until you're ready to feed it to your baby. The easiest way to remember storage guidelines for healthy full-term babies is the 4-4-6 rule. Simply put, your breast milk is okay at room temperature for up to four hours and can be stored in a clean BPA-free container or breast milk storage bag for up to four days in the coldest part of your refrigerator and in the freezer for up to six months. It's also a good idea to store your breast milk in quantities of 2 to 3 ounces to limit wasting your milk after it has been thawed. Keep in mind that thawed milk should be fed to your baby within 24 hours.

For a more comprehensive guide, see the human milk storage chart included (also in Appendix A), that was adapted from the Centers for Disease Control and Prevention (CDC) guidelines.

Human Milk Storage Guidelines (2019 CDC guidelines for healthy full-term babies)			
	Storage Location and Temperatures		
Type of Breastmilk	Countertop 77°F (25°C) or colder (room temperature)	Refrigerator 40°F (4°C)	Freezer 0°F (-18°C) or colder
Freshly Expressed or Pumped	Up to 4 Hours	Up to 4 Days	Within 6 months is best Up to 12 months is acceptable
Thawed, Previously Frozen	1 to 2 Hours	Up to 1 Day (24 hours)	NEVER refreeze human milk after it has been thawed
Leftover from a Feeding	Use within 2 hours after the baby is finished feeding		

CHAPTER 5: **Breastfeeding & Bottle Feeding** 73

Formula Feeding

How to Prepare Formula

Although preparing formula may seem like a no brainer, one thing that many parents don't realize is that they should be using water that has been boiled to at least 70°C or 158°F for mixing with powdered formula. Why do you ask? Powdered formula isn't sterile, and this step is to avoid the potential that your baby ingests harmful bacteria. Another critical thing to note is that after mixing the hot water with the powdered formula, you'll need to cool the mixture down. [10] For a detailed guide, see Appendix A.

The next important point is that you should adhere to the 2:1 mixture ratio, which is standard for most healthy full-term babies. Attempting to dilute formula (or add more water than recommended) could have dangerous consequences such as seizures. Adding too much powder to the formula mixture can be just as harmful and make your baby ill.

How much and how often should you feed your baby?

According to the American Academy of Pediatrics (2018), you should plan to feed your baby every 2 to 3 hours, within 24 hours, in the early weeks. Below you'll find some ranges to consider for the average amount of formula that healthy full-term babies drink during each bottle feeding.

Keep in mind that this is just a guide and may vary because no two babies are the same. As with any decisions about your baby's care or nutrition, you should discuss your baby's situation and nutritional needs with his or her pediatrician:

- *In the first couple of days after birth:* newborns drink around ½ ounce each feeding, with an increase of up to 1 to 2 oz by the time they're 3 to 5 days old. [11]
- *In the first couple of weeks:* 2 to 3 ounces (60 to 90 mL) of formula per feeding. [11]
- *By the end of the second month:* Your baby will be up to at least 4 to 5 ounces (120 mL), with a little more time in between feedings, amounting to around 6 to 8 feedings per day. [11]
- *At four months old:* babies drink up to 5 ounces per feeding. [11]
- *By 6 months:* Your baby will likely consume 6 to 8 ounces (180 to 240 mL). [11]

CHAPTER 6

Infant Safety & Health

"Making the decision to have a child - it is momentous. It is to decide forever to have your heart go walking around outside your body."

—Elizabeth Stone

In my neonatal intensive care unit (NICU) nursing days, we educated every caregiver on how to perform infant CPR, also known as cardiopulmonary resuscitation. Additionally, we showed parents how to feed their babies and performed a "car seat test." This test ensured that babies who were born too early (premature) would be able to breathe easily and safely during the car ride home. You may say, well duh, of course, those parents needed the additional training since their babies required specialized medical care and stayed in the hospital for weeks and sometimes months. Honestly, I suggest that all parents take an infant CPR class and learn all about the basic care of their baby and the safety measures that they should take once they're home. Education is so important, and learning about infant health and safety could save the life of your baby. Who knows, you may just happen to be in the right place at the right time to help someone else and save their baby's life.

In the United States of America (USA), the unfortunate truth is that the death of babies before their first birthday is far too high. In 2018, the infant mortality rate in the USA almost topped 6 deaths per 1,000 live births. The five leading causes of infant death in 2017 were: Birth defects, prematurity, low birth weight, maternal pregnancy-related complications, sudden infant death syndrome (SIDS), and injuries. For this chapter's purposes, I'll focus on the causes of death that occur after birth, which includes SIDS and injuries. [12]

The Nitty Gritty on Infant Safety

Car Seat Safety

A car seat is one of the single most important items that you will need to decide on for your baby. As a former NICU nurse, I have years of hands-on experience with car seats and know the most trusted brands like the back of my hand.

First and foremost, as always, do your research! Look into brands that may be suitable for your car model and type. Looking into safety ratings is a must and being familiar with your car seat is of the utmost importance. So please, I repeat, please don't show up to the labor & delivery unit with your car seat in a box and expect the nurses to help you put it together because, for liability reasons, this is something they almost always cannot do. If you're lucky, there may be a certified Child Passenger Safety Technician (CPST) working at the hospital who can assist you or answer your questions, but there is no guarantee.

I would strongly recommend researching how to schedule an appointment at a local Child Safety Seat Inspection Station (this is sometimes done at your local fire station, depending on where you live). This will ensure that a professional trained in car seat safety can help you get your seat correctly installed into your vehicle. After all, if you were ever in a car accident, you would never want to take the chance that your most precious cargo wasn't secured properly. Also, you will want to be sure to check for any potential safety recalls.

Last but not least, if you're considering using a used car seat or a "hand me down" from a friend, check the sticker on the side of the seat to ensure that the manufacture date is less than 10 years old. Another important note is that if you cannot verify without a shadow of a doubt that the seat has never been in a car accident, then you shouldn't consider using it at all. Again, this is your most precious bundle of joy we're talking about. For more information on car seat safety, see Appendix A.

Sudden Infant Death Syndrome (SIDS)

Even after a complete medical review and investigation, sudden infant death syndrome (SIDS) is the unexplained death of a baby before turning one year old. One of the proven ways to help decrease the occurrence of SIDS is to ensure that your baby is sleeping in a safe sleep environment and placed on his or her back. As always, you know I'm bringing the evidence-based information, so don't just take it from me; take a look at the following recommendations straight from the American Academy of Pediatrics (AAP) on infant sleep safety [13]:

- Until their first birthday, babies should be laid down to sleep on their backs, during naps, and at bedtime.
- Use a firm sleep surface.
- Room share — keeping your baby's sleep area in the same room where you sleep for the first six months minimally, but ideally for the first year.
- Never place your baby to sleep on a couch, sofa, or armchair. This is a dangerous place for your baby to sleep because he or she could suffocate (think loose pillows and seat cushions) or roll onto the floor.
- Bed-sharing is not recommended. Only bring your baby into your bed to feed or comfort.
- Keep bedding or any objects that could increase the risk of entrapment, suffocation, or strangulation out of the baby's sleep area.

Crib Safety

Long gone are the days of decorating the inside of your baby's crib with bumpers, stuffed animals, and comforters, or at least they should be by now. If this is news to you, please keep in mind that all of the items mentioned above pose a risk for suffocation or a situation where your baby may become "trapped," which could lead to cutting off their oxygen supply and prove to be deadly. I know that's heavy to read, but I have to keep it real with you and let you know how to keep your baby safe to allow him or her to live to their full potential, which is what I'm sure you want more than anything as a parent.

There are a few general guidelines for crib safety that I want to make sure you're aware of (see Appendix A for more information):

The wooden slats on your crib should be no more than 2³/₈ inches apart [14].

- In addition to the crib mattress being firm, it should fit snugly into the crib and not allow for any space in between the slats and the mattress [14].
- Always keep the sides of the crib raised to ensure that your baby cannot fall out.
- Ensure that you check for recalls on crib manufacturers before purchasing one.
- Try to stick to cribs that are relatively new without any visible wear and tear. If you decide to consider a "hand me down" or used crib and cannot confirm the crib's history, including manufacturer name, date, and recall history, it's probably a good idea to pass on it.
- If you're having trouble affording a crib, many non-profit organizations, churches, or your local birthing hospital may have resources to help you.

Choking, CPR, & First Aid

Choking Risks and Signs

Several choking hazards come to mind when I think about babies, and I'd like to make you aware of them so that you can avoid potential incidents.

These are some signs that your baby may be choking:

- There is unexplained coughing, especially during or after feedings.
- The baby's color turns from pink to blue. On darker-skinned babies looking at the lip color is usually the best indicator to tell if there is a color change.
- Your baby is having difficulty crying or unable to make any noise or cooing sounds.
- Noisy breathing.
- The baby appears to be struggling to breathe, which is usually evidenced by nostrils flaring or "pulling" noted around the throat or rib cage area (the medical term is retractions).

Choking Hazards and Risks

First up is choking that can occur from bottle propping. Bottle propping is the act of using an object like blankets, stuffed animals, or even a surface like the side of your baby's crib or swing to hold a bottle in place so that it doesn't need to be held by an adult. I'd like you to keep in mind that feeding your baby can be a great time to bond with your baby

CHAPTER 6: **Infant Safety & Health**

and look into his or her eyes. It can also be another excellent opportunity for you or your partner to hold your baby or do skin-to-skin. The big takeaway is that bottle propping of any type can prove to be dangerous.

Back in Chapter 5, I talked a lot about paced bottle feeding and why it's so important, but it's also a safer way to feed your baby because you are helping to control the flow of formula or breast milk that your baby is getting. Controlling the milk flow and ensuring that it isn't flowing from the bottle into your baby's mouth too fast is very important to help prevent your baby from choking.

Next is choking that can occur from putting solid foods or anything other than formula or breast milk into your baby's bottle. It's time for me to pull out the dramatics again because this is one of my pet peeves in infant safety, which is the idea that babies should be fed any other food in a bottle outside of formula or breast milk. It doesn't matter if your grandmother, favorite aunt, mommy friends, your mother, or mother-in-law tells you it's okay to dump a few tablespoons of rice cereal, oatmeal, or baby food into the bottle. Please, I repeat, please don't do it! All of the above are outdated practices and could cause your baby to choke even if you were told to just cut a "bigger hole" into the nipple so that the baby can drink it out of the bottle easier.

Also, think about older siblings or children who may be around your baby and not understand that babies cannot eat solid food or play with small toys.

If the sibling is old enough to understand simple explanations, it's always a great idea to begin talking with them about what is safe for babies and what can hurt them. Using basic easy to understand terms and even demonstrations can help get the point across with some repetition.

The takeaway here is to always remain aware and not leave your baby unattended. A baby monitor is not a replacement for you being attentive to your baby, but it is a good tool to have. A baby monitor or a similar phone app allows you to have eyes on your baby after placing him or her in the safety of their crib if you must leave the room where they're sleeping.

Why Should You Learn CPR?

CPR stands for cardiopulmonary resuscitation. A mouthful, I know. Although you may not be a medical professional or have never taken a CPR class in your life, doing so before you have your baby is a great idea. If you happen to get the advice about taking a CPR class after your baby is born, don't sweat it because there's no time like the present.

Learning the basics of CPR could potentially save a life because emergencies usually happen when we least expect them. Most infant CPR classes will teach you how to do chest compressions if needed, accident prevention, basic first aid, and what to do if your baby is choking.

If possible, I recommend taking an in-person class if one is available to you. Usually, classes are taught by a healthcare professional, like a nurse, and are typically offered at your local hospital. You can also find a private instructor through the American Heart Association (AHA) website or by asking your child's pediatrician or PNP (remember that's a pediatric nurse practitioner like me) for a recommendation.

I teach infant safety classes, virtually or in-person, that include a discussion of basic CPR and choking for infants, along with some of the other safety topics discussed in this chapter. Current technological advances make it much easier to accommodate busy families or those who may not have local access. Many instructors now offer an online or virtual option, an alternative to still get the education you need.

Injuries

Fall Prevention

Since this book is mostly about babies who are too young to be mobile, you may be wondering why on earth I need to discuss falls. The fact of the matter is that this is more of a public service announcement to be mindful that accidents can happen. So please never leave your baby unattended; on a bed, changing table, or on any piece of furniture that isn't a safe sleeping surface, like a crib. If your child does happen to take a tumble or fall, make sure they're not visibly hurt.

Next, you'll want to ensure that they're at a normal level of consciousness (awake and alert) and contact your healthcare provider for further advice. Of course, if a severe injury were to occur due to the fall, you should immediately call 911.

The Nitty Gritty on Infant Health

Immunizations

To vaccinate or to not vaccinate? Nowadays, there are so many opinions about whether or not parents should vaccinate their children. However, as I've mentioned before, opinions are just that, so I challenge you to do your research and be informed in your decision. As a pediatric nurse practitioner, I highly recommend that all the families I work with vaccinate their children.

The evidence is clear that vaccines help keep life-threatening diseases at bay and help to keep your child healthier in the long run, and offer some protection to children and people with weakened immune systems. According to the World Health Organization (WHO), "vaccination is one of the most effective ways to prevent diseases. A vaccine helps the body's immune system recognize and fight pathogens like viruses or bacteria, which keeps us safe from the diseases they cause. [15]

Timing of Immunizations (aka "shots")

It is highly recommended that you follow the Centers for Disease Control and Prevention's (CDC) immunization schedule for infants and children (see Appendix A). This is usually the schedule most pediatric healthcare providers who practice evidence-based care follow. Your child's age, type of vaccine, and the recommendations for the frequency your child would need the immunization are listed. However, when advising you on the vaccines that your child will need, their health history will need to be considered. The first vaccine that your child typically receives after he or she is born, with your consent, of course, is the hepatitis B vaccine.

I strongly recommend that you follow the CDC immunization schedule, but if you decide that you must delay or space out vaccines for any reason, then you should plan to discuss this with your pediatrician. Remember that you'll want to discuss any policies that your child's healthcare provider may have when vaccines are concerned before selecting them to manage your child's care. This is very important to do when deciding on a pediatrician or PNP to take care of your baby. Some pediatric offices may have stricter policies than others to follow evidence-based guidelines and protect themselves, office staff, and any other people they may come in contact with, including their own families.

Medical Emergencies

You'll find a brief list of some common medical emergencies in addition to those discussed earlier in this chapter, in the section on CPR. Also, you'll always want to have the poison control phone number handy for yourself or any caregiver of your baby, should any hazardous or poisonous items be accidentally swallowed, touched, or get into your little one's eyes. An excellent place to keep the number is saved in your phone contacts or somewhere in plain view, like on the front of your refrigerator. You can reach the poison control helpline by calling 1-800-222-1222.

Although all the potential emergencies that could occur aren't listed, below, you'll find a helpful reference for you to begin discussions with your child's healthcare provider so that you're better prepared should any of these situations ever occur. I know it's easier said than done, but always try to remain calm.

Every situation listed below would be a reason to reach out to your baby's licensed healthcare provider or call 911 immediately.

- Fever in any baby under 3 months is always an emergency and, frankly, a pretty big deal. A fever is defined at 100.4°F temperature. In small babies, temperatures should be taken rectally. As they get older, you can start taking them carefully underneath the arm (armpit area). Make sure that you always have a working thermometer that you're familiar with using in your home.

- Seizures are always considered an emergency and can occur for many reasons in infants. One of the most common is a seizure that occurs due to your baby's body temperature rising to a dangerously low or high level. Seizures usually result in shaking, trembling, or jerking movements. However, seizures can also present as a dazed look or unresponsiveness, especially in older children.

- Vomiting that doesn't stop and shoots out of your baby's mouth forcefully. This becomes a bigger deal when your baby cannot keep down formula or breast milk after drinking it, especially when diarrhea is also a factor. Note: Diarrhea shouldn't be confused with the typical thin, seedy, mustard-colored stools commonly seen in breastfed infants mentioned in Chapter 3.

CHAPTER 7

Explaining Facts vs. Myths

*"Motherhood is the greatest thing
and the hardest thing."*

—Ricki Lake

Nicole is one of my more memorable clients from when I first began my private lactation practice. Not only was she funny, but her baby Kyle, who was 6 months at the time, was the absolute cutest! Nicole came to me for a return to work consultation, which is where I help moms plan a strategy to continue breastfeeding their baby after they transition back to work at the end of their maternity leave. I worked with Nicole virtually, so we met via secure video software, and we reviewed all of her questions and came up with a plan that would fit into her work schedule and lifestyle. So by now, you're thinking that sounds totally normal and routine, except poor Nicole had been told by her grandmother that she should add some rice cereal to baby Kyle's bottle to help him sleep through the night, so she could get more rest in preparation for work the next day. Nicole tried adding the cereal to baby Kyle's bottles for around a week and noticed that he became constipated and seemed fussier than usual after feedings.

So why am I telling you this story? Well, because the advice that Nicole received from her grandmother isn't all that uncommon. In fact, myself as a new mother and many of the families that I've worked with, have been given the same advice. Honestly, there's no evidence to support that offering rice cereal or any solids for that matter will help your baby sleep longer at night. A 2010 study found that although feeding a baby solid foods may lead to fewer feedings at night, it didn't necessarily decrease the number of times babies wake at night. [16] Not to mention, as discussed back in Chapter 6, adding any additional solids to your baby's bottle can be a choking hazard or lead to digestive issues.

You learn some things in life from experience and trial and error, but if you have accurate, evidence-based information at your fingertips, why not use it to weed out the myths, aka "fake news"?

To provide parents with some options to find trustworthy information, my website has a resource list that includes links to parenting, child health, breastfeeding, and mental health websites. Additionally, in Appendix A, you'll find a great list of evidence-based resources readily available to refer back to at any time.

Common Myths Versus Facts

For some strange reason, there seem to be so many myths behind feeding infants. Could it be the whole ESP (remember that means eat, sleep, poop) factor? Since eating is such a significant part of a baby's life and their growth and development depend so much upon it, parents research this topic a lot.

Unfortunately, much of the time, parents find a ton of unsolicited or poor advice. Below I've created a list of some of the most common myths I've heard over the last decade, broken down by topic.

Myths About Feeding Your Baby

Myth: Breastfeeding is painful.

Fact: Although in the early days, breastfeeding can be uncomfortable or lead to sore nipples, in general, it shouldn't be painful. Painful breastfeeding often signifies that you and your baby may need some help with proper latch and positioning techniques or to schedule an appointment with a lactation professional.

Myth: Your baby can be allergic to your breast milk.

Fact: Babies are not allergic to their mom's breast milk but may have a cow's milk or soy protein intolerance. Some of the most common signs and symptoms include bloody stools, skin rashes (also known as eczema), excessive fussiness, and upset stomach (also known as reflux). If you feel your baby may be suffering from a combination of these symptoms, keep a daily food diary to track what you're eating and discuss any potential issues with your child's healthcare provider.

I personally lived this experience with my son when I found out that he had a dairy and soy intolerance when he was around 2 months old. I know how tough it can be to eliminate familiar foods from your diet and find adequate support. Two helpful tips that I'd like to share are that you can find countless delicious dairy-free recipe ideas on Pinterest and that there a quite a few helpful support groups on Facebook, believe it or not. See Appendix A for a list of resources.

Myth: If you're breastfeeding, you shouldn't drink coffee.

Fact: Coffee, when consumed within reason, doesn't show evidence of being unsafe for breastfeeding mothers' babies. What we do know is that drinking an excessive amount, like more than five cups a day, can cause some babies to become jittery, irritable, and negatively affect their sleep. Let's be honest; no one should probably be drinking more than five cups of anything that's not water. However, if you'd like to be extra careful, keep in mind that caffeine levels usually peak in the body, meaning they're at the highest level around one hour after consumption. [17] So this isn't a memo to go out and guzzle down a whole pot of coffee, but it reveals that you can at least enjoy a cup of coffee while breastfeeding. As with anything related to you or your baby's health, you should always consult with your healthcare provider or pediatrician.

Myth: If you're breastfeeding, you should never drink an alcoholic beverage.

Fact: Moderation is essential when you're considering drinking alcohol as a breastfeeding mother. Generally speaking, having 1 to 2 drinks will not be harmful to your baby but having said that, every person's body breaks down alcohol differently based on genetics and weight. The bottom line is, you can have a drink or two while breastfeeding. However, you should weigh the risks, as with anything, which could be a short-term decrease in your milk supply, the fact that your baby may seem more agitated, or that his or her baseline sleep patterns may be negatively impacted.

According to research, waiting for an average of 2 to 2½ hours in between drinking an alcoholic drink and nursing your baby may help to decrease any adverse effects. In summary, having a drink or two will most likely not hurt your baby, and you don't have to "pump and dump" your milk, which is a common misconception. [18]

Myth: Oatmeal or sports drinks will increase your breast milk supply.

Fact: This is more of a half-truth rather than utterly false because although some mothers may perceive an increase in their breast milk supply after they drink sports drinks or eat oatmeal, there's no scientific evidence of this being true. Generally speaking, no food, drink, or pill alone will result in you having a plentiful milk supply. The key is to try to work with a lactation professional to understand if and why your milk supply is low and to express milk from your breasts frequently (every 2 to 3 hours) by latching your baby, hand expressing, or pumping.

Sometimes herbal supplements can be considered but should always be discussed with your healthcare provider, in addition to deciding if potential benefits in your particular situation outweigh the potential side effects. A great resource to read more about this topic is kellymom.com. I also recommend discussing this with an IBCLC.

Myths About Illness
Myth: Teething causes a fever.
Fact: Not true, not true, not true! Yes, I needed to say it that many times to make sure you get the point. I have literally had people try to argue this point, and dare I repeat it again, it's just not true. Frequently, when babies are teething, you may find that they have their hands or other objects in their mouth, which could introduce him or her to germs, and germs lead to fever, not teething. So that is one potential correlation between teething and fever, especially in mobile babies. As a reminder, back in Chapter 6, I mentioned that a fever (100.4°F) in any baby three months or less is a medical emergency until proven otherwise.

Myths About Comforting Your Baby

Myth: If you hold your baby too much or respond whenever they cry, you will spoil them.

Fact: This is absolutely false! Way back in the day, a psychologist named Erik Erikson introduced theories related to infant development. He highlighted studies that explained that when parents meet their baby's basic needs early on by providing affection and a safe, secure environment, it leads to a trusting and loving relationship between parent and child. On the other hand, not meeting some of these basic but essential needs leads to the absence of a trusting relationship between parent and child. [19] As parents, it is our job to nurture and care for our babies, and responding to their needs, which are often communicated by crying, is part of that. Honestly, the opportunity to hold your baby won't always be there as they grow and establish more independence, so try to take advantage of it while you can, especially in the early months and years.

Myths About Your Baby's Development

Myth: Babies who use walkers will walk at an earlier age.

Fact: Again, this is false, and honestly, infant walkers are not recommended because they can become a safety hazard, especially if you live in a home with steps or one that has not been baby-proofed.

CHAPTER 8

Sleep & Developmental Milestones

"If your baby is beautiful and perfect, never cries or fusses, sleeps on schedule and burps on demand, an angel all the time, you're the grandma."

—THERESA BLOOMINGDALE

Oh, sleep that sweet, sweet "S" word that all parents are craving, and some would literally give anything for. Trust me, I understand. Like I really understand! It took nearly 2 years for my husband and I to get our son to sleep through the night in his own crib.

But let's get back to this chapter's point, which is for me to discuss what you can really expect as far as sleep is concerned in the first three months (also known as the fourth trimester). Unfortunately, it won't involve a magical solution where I tell you that you can get your baby to sleep through the night in a week. Instead, it's my goal to help you set realistic sleep expectations.

Okay, now brace yourself as I tell you what the average "full night of sleep" actually is for a newborn. The answer is 2½ to 4 hours, yes 2½ to 4 hours! [20] I'm repeating it so that

I can help you to understand that if your newborn baby is gaining weight appropriately and sleeping for up to four hours at a time, you should start celebrating because four hours is a nice stretch of sleep for a newborn.

On the other end of the spectrum, it's also normal if your baby is still waking at night during the first month or even twelve months. Is this fun? No. Does it make for sleepy parents? Yes. However, there are so many normal ranges on the infant sleep scale that I just want to make sure you're not being too hard on yourself if your baby is not quite there yet.

Normal Sleep Cycles

Newborn Sleep

I've talked about sleep expectations some, so I want to dive a little deeper into what can be considered normal. First, what does normal really mean? I honestly don't care to use the word because, in general, there are many variations of what regular sleep cycles can look like for babies. On average, a healthy newborn baby would be expected to sleep between 16 to 18 hours per day. [20] Does this mean your baby will sleep 16 consecutive hours in a row? Certainly not. I think I already deflated that dream when I discussed realistic expectations with you. During the span of a 24 hour day, the amount of sleep that your baby gets can be somewhat inconsistent because newborn babies have no concept of day versus night. Let's face it, they have a mind of their own and may only sleep for one to two hours at a time.

CHAPTER 8: **Sleep & Developmental Milestones**

Infant Sleep

From around 4 months to 12 months of age, babies should sleep between 12 to 16 hours each day to help support proper development and growth. [21]

The older your baby gets, the more daytime/nighttime confusion lessens, and sleeping overnight usually happens in more consecutive hours. By six months old, most babies can sleep up to 6 hours or more in a row. [21] Your baby will typically need around two naps per day as well.

Sleep Guidance and Tips

I explained the typical amount of sleeping hours that your baby needs and how to manage your expectations so that you don't fall into the "why won't my baby sleep?" trap that can drain your joy as a parent. Know that the phase where sleep hours and lengths are inconsistent is usually just that— a phase.

Before the age of 6 months, sleep training your baby is something I strongly recommend against, based on available research and what is known to be true about typical sleep patterns in young babies. Many methods exist, but I caution you to do your research, and if something doesn't seem or feel right, you shouldn't do it. Even if your best friend said it worked for her three children. Also, consider that babies usually cry for a reason. Based on the trust versus mistrust theory that I discussed in Chapter 7, as a parent, you want to do your best to nurture and ensure that your baby feels cared for and safe.

So on with the tips! One of the most important things you'll want to consider is a routine for your baby and one that will be realistic for you to maintain. Don't worry; routines can be altered if they don't work well, but it's best to remain as consistent as possible. The purpose behind being consistent is to help prepare your baby for sleep each night.

- The routine should happen around the same time each evening.
- Some things that you may find helpful are a warm bath, storytime, playing soft music, singing lullabies, quiet time spent cuddling, and breastfeeding or bottle feeding.
- You may need to add in some additional bottle or breastfeeding sessions for babies in the early weeks and months should they wake at night to help maintain their weight gain or just because they wake up hungry.

Consider Temperament and Personality

Many times, parents envision that their baby will be just like the babies in the movies. You know the ones that cry and sleep on cue. But the truth is that your baby's personality or temperament can vary. The best experience will be getting to know your little one and how to best care for and meet his or her needs.

For babies, temperaments can span from the perfect little angel to "not so perfect." **The three most common behaviors are:**

1. The "easy child" accounts for a little under half of all children who usually follow a pretty predictable schedule for ESP (remember that means eating, sleeping, and pooping), adapts well to changes in routine, people, or environment. Overall, he or she will have an easy-going disposition. [22]

2. The "difficult child" accounts for around 10% of children who don't follow a predictable ESP pattern, don't react well to new stimuli, and can be, dare I say, a little cranky and hard to adjust at times. [22]

3. The "slow to warm up child" accounts for 15% of the infant and child population and includes those who usually aren't very active, avoid new situations and encounters, take a while to adjust, and can be somewhat cranky or perceived as having negative attitudes. [22]

So why do temperaments even matter? Well, plain and simple, it is essential to know that all children aren't the same and that variations in personality type can occur even amongst siblings. Hence, as a pediatric healthcare provider, I just want you to be aware that your parenting style may vary based on your child's temperament and personality. This is likely one reason why some of the "it worked for me" advice from friends or family may not be a good fit for you. It's best to get to know your baby and adapt your parenting style based on what they need and how they best receive your love, nurturing, and care.

Purple Crying

Did you know that many babies go through a period of crying a lot and that it's totally normal? A term that I want you to be familiar with is purple crying. Developed by the National Center on Shaken Baby Syndrome is the Period of PURPLE Crying®. A research-based education program that teaches parents about the normal (see that word again) period of heightened crying that many parents experience with their babies. Even though PURPLE crying is seen in most babies, the degree to which it happens can vary from very mild to pretty intense in duration and intensity for some. [23] (see Appendix A)

The acronym **PURPLE** stands for:

- **P**eak of crying
- **U**nexpected
- **R**esists soothing
- **P**ain-like face
- **L**ong-lasting
- **E**vening

You may be asking yourself what this all means, so here is a summary of what to look out for:

- Crying that lasts for more than 6 hours a day.
- By two months old, crying can peak.

- Your baby may not be easy to calm despite your best efforts.
- Crying may leave you feeling distressed or just plain tapped out.
- Crying may be worse later on in the day.
- Your baby may seem like he or she is in pain.

If there's one essential thing to note, crying is normal even though it can lead to frustration. It's okay to be at your wit's end but please never, ever shake your baby. My best advice is if you ever find yourself in a state of anger or feel like you just cannot deal, then be sure to place your baby in a safe location within the eye's view, like their crib. Then, after your baby is safe and secure, take a few minutes to take some deep long breaths in and out to regain your calm. You may even find screaming into a pillow to be therapeutic.

Infant Development
Normal Development

Chances are that if you've been around a nurse or doctor, you have heard us say "it depends" in response to a question about what is typical in terms of development, and the truth of the matter is that it really does depend. The variations of what can be considered within an acceptable range for most babies at a certain age or developmental stage are pretty vast.

Your child's healthcare provider should also be asking you questions during each well-child visit to screen your child and note any red flags that may require early intervention services. For this chapter's purpose, I'll stick with the first 6 months of developmental milestones to give you a good idea of how you should expect your baby to be progressing. The following list was adapted from the 19th edition of *The Harriett Lane Handbook* [24]:

One-month milestones
- Your baby can raise his or her head while on their stomach.
- Can grasp your finger tightly.
- Reacts to sound.

Two-month milestones
- Lifts chest up from a flat surface.
- Follows object past midline (center of their body).
- Smiles socially, usually in response to voices or touch.
- Recognizes parent.

Three-month milestones
- Begins to hold head up steadily.
- Brings hands to mouth and can open and close them.
- Makes cooing sounds.

Four-month milestones
- Rolls over from front to back.
- Brings hands to the midline of their body.
- Laughs.
- Grasps toys.
- Enjoys looking around.

Six-month milestones
- Starts to sit without support.
- Transfers objects between hands.
- Babbles.
- Rolls over from front to back and back to front.
- Tries to grasp at objects within reach.
- Enjoys playing with familiar people.

Closing Thoughts

I hope that now that you've completed this book, you've learned some helpful tips about baby care and how to prepare for the postpartum period. Whether you've read this book as a new mother or a veteran mom of four, I want you to feel empowered to venture into motherhood with the knowledge of how to continue seeking out reliable resources that can add to your "motherhood toolkit." Remember that parenting is a never-ending journey of learning as you navigate through it. No matter what struggles you've encountered so far, you will survive and emerge as a confident mama! I'm sure of it!

So now what? It doesn't have to end here; I know I certainly don't want it to! I welcome you to join my Facebook and Instagram communities @mercedesthenp, check out the content, chat with me, and interact with the other parents as often as you like. Also, for more information about my parenting classes and be the first to know about future workshops and events, head over to *www.MercedesThomas.com*.

Acknowledgements

This book is a labor of love, and first and foremost, I would like to thank God for giving me the strength and endurance to complete this book during an unprecedented time that many of us lived through in 2020. To my husband AnJuan 'Juan' for his love and support and for allowing me the space to create and follow my dreams. To my son Ashton, the reason I decided to take this book from an idea that I had nearly a decade ago to a reality. Being his mother has shaped my practice as a nurse and the way that I'm able to empathize with and educate parents. And most of all, my mother because without her, there is no me; she is my role model, inspiration, and biggest cheerleader. Finally, I would like to thank my mentor Catie and coach Gertrude who offered their encouragement, and wisdom and my friend Odi who selflessly offered her advice and time to help me with the early stages of editing in the midst of being a busy nurse and entrepreneur.

APPENDIX A
Resources

Chapter 1:
Doulas
https://doulamatch.net/
https://www.dona.org
https://www.blackdoulas.org

Childbirth Education and Resources
www.lamaze.org
www.hypnobirthing.com/
https://evidencebasedbirth.com

Birth Plan
https://kidshealth.org/en/parents/birth-plans.html

Chapter 2:
Postpartum Mood and Anxiety Disorders
https://www.postpartum.net

Mental Health Resources
https://therapyforblackgirls.com/
https://www.psychologytoday.com/us

Mommy Mood Tracker™ (pdf version)
https://mailchi.mp/d66fb0ef78e1/mommymoodtracker

Chapter 3:
Baby-Friendly Hospitals
https://www.babyfriendlyusa.org/

Chapter 4:
The Fourth Trimester
https://newmomhealth.com/

Support Groups
https://www.babycafeusa.org/for-parents.html
https://www.postpartum.net/get-help/psi-online-support-meetings/

Chapter 5:
General Breastfeeding Information
www.kellymom.com
www.llli.org

Breastfeeding Videos
https://globalhealthmedia.org/videos/breastfeeding/

Donor Breast Milk
https://www.hmbana.org/
https://www.milkbank.org/

Find an IBCLC Near You
www.ilca.org

APPENDIX A: **Resources** 113

Medication Safety During Pregnancy and Lactation
https://www.infantrisk.com/

Hand Expression
https://firstdroplets.com/

Human Milk Storage and Preparation Guidelines
https://www.cdc.gov/breastfeeding/recommendations/handling_breastmilk.htm

Breastfeeding Laws in the Workplace
https://www.womenshealth.gov/supporting-nursing-moms-work

How to Safely Prepare Formula
https://www.who.int/foodsafety/document_centre/PIF_Bottle_en.pdf?ua=1

Chapter 6:
Car Seat Safety
https://www.nhtsa.gov

Safe Sleep for Infants
https://kidshealth.org/en/parents/sids.html

https://www.healthychildren.org/English/ages-stages/baby/sleep/Pages/Preventing-SIDS.aspx

Crib Safety & Recalls

https://safetosleep.nichd.nih.gov/resources/caregivers/environment/look

https://www.cpsc.gov/Safety-Education/Safety-Guides/Kids-and-Babies/Cribs/

Find a CPR Class

https://cpr.heart.org/en/course-catalog-search#whichcourse

Immunizations

https://www.who.int/vaccines/questions-and-answers

https://www.cdc.gov/vaccines/parents/schedules/index.html

Medical Emergencies

https://www.healthychildren.org/English/health-issues/injuries-emergencies/Pages/When-Your-Child-Needs-Emergency-Medical-Services.aspx

Poison Control

https://www.poison.org/

Chapter 7:
Milk Soy Protein Intolerance (CMPI)

http://infantproctocolitis.org/

Cow's Milk Protein Allergy (CMPA)

https://gikids.org/digestive-topics/cows-milk-protein-allergy/

https://kidshealth.org/en/parents/milk-allergy.html

Chapter 8:
Developmental Milestone Tools

https://www.cdc.gov/ncbddd/actearly/parents/index.html

Purple Crying

http://www.purplecrying.info/

APPENDIX B
References

1

DONA International (2018). *What is a Doula?* Retrieved July 20, 2020, from https://www.dona.org/what-is-a-doula/

2

American College of Obstetricians and Gynecologists (2018). *Optimizing postpartum care.* ACOG Committee Opinion No. 736. Obstet Gynecol;131:e140–150.

3

K. França, T. Rodrigues, J. Ledon, J. Savas and A. Chacon, "Comprehensive Overview and Treatment Update on Hair Loss," *Journal of Cosmetics, Dermatological Sciences and Applications,* Vol. 3 No. 3A, 2013, pp. 1-8. doi: 10.4236/jcdsa.2013.33A1001

4

American Pregnancy Association (2020). *Baby Blues.* Retrieved July 27, 2020, from https://american-pregnancy.org/first-year-of-life/baby-blues/

5

Centers for Disease Control and Prevention (2020) *Depression Among Women.* Retrieved July 27, 2020, from https://www.cdc.gov/reproductivehealth /depression/index.htm

6

Postpartum Support International (2020). *Pregnancy & Postpartum Mental Health Overview*. Retrieved June 30, 2020, from https://www.postpartum.net/learn-more/pregnancy-postpartum-mental-health/

7

World Health Organization (2020). *Breastfeeding*. Retrieved June 30, 2020, from https://www.who.int/health-topics/breastfeeding

8

American Academy of Pediatrics, Section on Breastfeeding. (2012). Breastfeeding and the Use of Human Milk. *Pediatrics*, 129(3), E827-E841. doi:10.1542/peds.2011-3552

9

Butte, N.F., Lopez-Alarcon, & Garza, C. (2002). *Nutrient Adequacy of Exclusive Breastfeeding for the Term Infant During the First Six Months of Life*. Geneva, Switzerland, World Health Organization.

10

Food and Agriculture Organization of the United Nations (FAO) and the World Health Organization (WHO) (2007). Safe Preparation, Storage and Handling of Powdered Infant Formula Guidelines. Retrieved August 20, 2020, from https://www.who.int/ foodsafety/publications/powdered-infant-formula/en/

11

Jain, S. (2018). How Often and How Much Should Your Baby Eat? Retrieved June 10, 2020, from https://www.healthychildren.org/English/ages-stages/baby/feeding-nutrition/Pages/How-Often-and-How-Much-Should-Your-Baby-Eat.aspx

12

Centers for Disease Control and Prevention. *Infant Mortality.* (2020, September 10). Retrieved July 1, 2020, from https://www.cdc.gov/reproductivehealth/maternalinfanthealth/infantmortality.htm

13

Moon, R. (2020, February 10). *How to Keep Your Sleeping Baby Safe: AAP Policy Explained.* Retrieved June 10, 2020, from https://www.healthychildren.org/English/agesstages/baby/sleep/Pages/A-ParentsGuide-to-SafeSleep.aspx

14

Hagan JF, Shaw JS, Duncan PM, eds. *Bright Futures: Guidelines for Health Supervision of Infants, Children, and Adolescents* [pocket guide]. 4th ed. Elk Grove Village, IL: American Academy of Pediatrics; 2017

15

World Health Organization (2020). *Vaccines and immunization.* Retrieved October 30, 2020, from https://www.who.int/topics/vaccines/en/

16

Brown, A., & Harries, V. (2015). Infant sleep and night feeding patterns during later infancy: association with breastfeeding frequency, daytime complementary food intake, and infant weight. *Breastfeeding medicine: the official journal of the Academy of Breastfeeding Medicine*, 10(5), 246–252. https://doi.org/10.1089/bfm.2014.0153

17

Drugs and Lactation Database (LactMed) [Internet]. Bethesda (MD): National Library of Medicine (US); 2006. Caffeine. [Updated 2019 Jun 30]. Available from: https://www.ncbi.nlm.nih.gov/ books/ NBK501467/

18

Drugs and Lactation Database (LactMed) [Internet]. Bethesda (MD): National Library of Medicine (US); 2006-. Alcohol. [Updated 2020 May 11]. Available from: https://www.ncbi.nlm.nih.gov/books/ NBK501469/

19

Orenstein GA, Lewis L. Erikson's Stages of Psychosocial Development. [Updated 2020 Mar 9]. In: StatPearls [Internet]. Treasure Island (FL): StatPearls Publishing; 2020 Jan. Available from: https://www.ncbi.nlm.nih.gov/books/ NBK556096/

APPENDIX B: **References** 121

20
Davis, K., Parker, K., & Montgomery, G. (March–April 2004). Sleep in infants and young Children Part one: Normal sleep. *Journal of Pediatric Health Care*. doi:10.1016/S0891-5245(03)00149-4.

21
Paruthi S, Brooks LJ, D'Ambrosio C, Hall WA, Kotagal S, Lloyd RM, Malow BA, Maski K, Nichols C, Quan SF, Rosen CL, Troester MM, Wise MS. Recommended amount of sleep for pediatric populations: a consensus statement of the American Academy of Sleep Medicine. *J Clin Sleep Med* 2016;12(6):785–786.

22
Behrman, R. E., Kliegman, R., Jenson, H. & Marcdante, K. (2011). *Nelson Essentials of Pediatrics*. Philadelphia, PA: Saunders/Elsevier.

23
Adam Miconi, R. (n.d.). What is the period of purple crying? Retrieved August 12, 2020, from http://purplecrying.info/what-is-the-period-of-purple-crying.php

24
Tschudy, M. M., & Arcara, K. M. (2012). *The Harriet Lane Handbook: a manual for pediatric house officers*. 19th ed. Philadelphia, PA: Mosby Elsevier.

Made in the USA
Coppell, TX
14 June 2022